LIBRARY
MILWAUKEE AREA TECHNIC
Milwaukee Campus

P9-ELU-282

100 Questions & Answers About Acne

DATE DUE

FE 19'08		
OCT 0 8 2008		

Demco, Inc. 38-293

616.53
D273

World Headquarters

Jones and Bartlett	Jones and Bartlett	Jones and Bartlett
Publishers	Publishers Canada	Publishers International
40 Tall Pine Drive	2406 Nikanna Road	Barb House, Barb Mews
Sudbury, MA 01776	Mississauga, ON L5C 2W6	London W6 7PA
info@jbpub.com	CANADA	UK
www.jbpub.com		

Copyright © 2005 by Jones and Bartlett Publishers, Inc.

All rights reserved. No part of the material protected by this copyright notice may be reproduced or utilized in any form, electronic or mechanical, including photocopying, recording, or by any information storage and retrieval system, without written permission from the copyright owner.

Library of Congress Cataloging-in-Publication Data

Day, Doris J.
 100 questions & answers about acne / Doris J. Day.-- 1st ed.
   p. cm.
 Includes index.
 ISBN 0-7637-4569-3 (pbk.)
 1. Acne--Popular works. I. Title: One hundred questions and answers about
acne. II. Title.
 RL131.D39 2005
 616.5'3--dc22
                                                    2004013093

The authors, editor, and publisher have made every effort to provide accurate information. However, they are not responsible for errors, omissions, or for any outcomes related to the use of the contents of this book and take no responsibility for the use of the products described. Treatments and side effects described in this book may not be applicable to all patients; likewise, some patients may require a dose or experience a side effect that is not described herein. The reader should confer with his or her own physician regarding specific treatments and side effects. Drugs and medical devices are discussed that may have limited availability controlled by the Food and Drug Administration (FDA) for use only in a research study or clinical trial. The drug information presented has been derived from reference sources, recently published data, and pharmaceutical tests. Research, clinical practice, and government regulations often change the accepted standard in this field. When consideration is being given to use of any drug in the clinical setting, the health care provider or reader is responsible for determining FDA status of the drug, reading the package insert, reviewing prescribing information for the most up-to-date recommendations on dose, precautions, and contraindications, and determining the appropriate usage for the product. This is especially important in the case of drugs that are new or seldom used. The statements of the patients quoted in this book represent their own opinions and do not necessarily reflect the views of the authors or the publisher.

PRODUCTION CREDITS
Chief Executive Officer: Clayton Jones
Chief Operating Officer: Don W. Jones, Jr.
President, Higher Education and Professional Publishing: Robert W. Holland, Jr.
V.P., Sales and Marketing: William J. Kane
V.P., Design and Production: Anne Spencer
V.P., Manufacturing and Inventory Control: Therese Bräuer
Executive Publisher: Christopher Davis
Special Projects Editor: Elizabeth Platt
Editorial Assistant: Kathy Richardson
Marketing Manager: Matthew Payne
Text Design: Kristin Ohlin
Cover Design: Philip Regan
Composition: Northeast Compositors, Inc.
Text and Cover Printing: Malloy, Inc.

Printed in the United States of America
08 07 06 05 04   10 9 8 7 6 5 4 3 2 1

Contents

Introduction   v

Part 1. Acne Overview   1

Questions 1–19 describe basic facts about acne:
- What is acne?
- Who gets acne?
- What causes acne?

Part 2. Acne Myths and Facts   43

Questions 20–31 address common misconceptions and highlights underlying causes of acne, such as:
- Does chocolate cause acne?
- Can greasy food or any food cause or make acne worse?
- Does dirty skin make acne worse?

Part 3. When to Treat   63

Questions 32–37 discuss factors to consider when thinking about treatment, including:
- I get only a few pimples each month. Do I need to treat them?
- Why do I always get acne in the same spots?
- Do I need a blood test to evaluate my acne?

Part 4. Topical Acne Treatment   73

Questions 38–55 discuss the types and availability of various topical treatments, including:
- What different types of topical treatments are available for acne?
- How long should it take to see results?
- Why are there so many different treatments for acne?

Part 5. Oral Antibiotics   103

Questions 56–65 review considerations for the use of oral antibiotics, such as:
- When should I consider taking oral antibiotics?

- If I take an oral antibiotic, will it make me resistant to antibiotics if I really need to take them at a later time?
- What are the most common side effects of oral antibiotics?

Part 6. Oral Isotretinoin   119

Questions 66–78 discuss the use of isotretinoin as treatment for acne:
- What is oral isotretinoin?
- Am I a good candidate for oral isotretinoin?
- How does isotretinoin work?

Part 7. Hormonal Treatments   137

Questions 79–82 describe hormonal therapies for acne, including:
- What is hormonal therapy? Do I need to have my hormones evaluated?
- What hormonal therapy is right for me?
- Does every oral contraceptive help acne?

Part 8. Procedures Done in the Doctor's Office   149

Questions 83–94 detail surgical and other procedures to treat acne and acne scars, including:
- What procedures can be used to treat acne?
- Are chemical peels safe?
- What is dermabrasion?

Part 9. Other Treatments/Experimental Methods   163

Questions 95–100 address alternative and experimental treatments for acne, such as:
- Are herbal supplements safe for acne? Do they work for acne?
- How does photodynamic therapy work?
- How do I know if a treatment I heard about in the media will work?

Appendix   169

The Appendix contains a list of organizations, print resources, and Web sites to help people with acne to find more information about treatment.

Glossary   171

Index   177

Smooth, flawless skin—it is what we all strive for. It is perfection itself. It defines beauty, exudes confidence, and implies success. Acne is an obstacle to beautiful skin. It distorts the otherwise smooth contour; leaves the skin red, bumpy, and uneven in tone; and leaves behind scars that can last a lifetime. It makes people feel embarrassed and self-conscious. It creates a barrier between the beauty within and the face that we put forward. The good news is that, if treated early and appropriately, it can be controlled so that the negative impact is minimized or, ideally, completely erased.

The skin is our largest and, I would offer, most beautiful organ. We cannot exist without it; however, unlike other essential organs such as the heart or kidneys, which cannot replace themselves if damaged, the skin is designed to intentionally replace and renew itself regularly. This is clearly an advantage in that the constant turnover allows for damage to the skin to be corrected and to keep the skin looking refreshed and renewed. It is very important to keep our skin healthy and intact in order to both look our best and avoid deeper problems.

Conveniently located on the outside of our body, the skin serves many vital functions that are essential for life. It creates a barrier protecting our internal organs from the ravages of the outside world. It protects us against infection and even has its own special network of circulating protective cells called Langerhans cells, which offer a very important first line of defense. The skin is also the major organ that helps maintain and regulate body temperature and water balance. Constant adjustments are made in the skin and through the skin that remove certain toxins that our body has created.

On a deeper level, the skin has touch receptors that help us sense pain and thus avoid damage from burns or excessive force or other harmful elements. Those same touch receptors in the skin allow us to experience maximal pleasure and express love.

The skin also serves a very important aesthetic function. How we perceive and project ourselves to others is based largely on how we think we look, which is based largely on how our skin looks. Ideal skin has a smooth, even complexion with no obvious pores; it is also supple and wrinkle free. Of course, this ideal exists only on the covers of magazines, where exceedingly thin, airbrushed models tease us into believing that such goals are truly attainable when in reality they are only figments of our collective imagination and marketing agency talents.

Getting our skin to look good and keeping it that way have become a multibillion dollar per year industry, and it affects us to our deepest core. Virtually hundreds of thousands of products are available that claim to be the latest, newest, and best product to give you flawless skin that will change your life overnight. We are all always looking for the newest, secret, magical ingredient that will clear any problems in our skin, real or imagined, from acne to wrinkles, and give us that "glow" that signals health, beauty, youth, and success.

Acne is a condition of the skin that is more than just about how we look: It can also be a sign of, or be made worse by, hormonal disturbance, stress, medications, or other factors. The scarring that can result from even mild acne can last a lifetime and serves as a painful reminder of the acne that was.

Acne is the most common skin disorder in the United States, affecting over 17 million people. It can be a debilitating, scarring, disfiguring condition that can affect anyone of any age, gender, or ethnicity at any time. Many myths about acne exist that make it even more difficult for some people to manage and understand their condition. For example, many people think that acne is just for teenagers and that they just have to put up with it or hide or cover it up as best they can until they outgrow it. The truth is that acne can occur at any age, and because of its potential for scarring, it should be treated and controlled from its early onset. Also, many people do not outgrow their acne and require regular or intermittent treatment, sometimes indefinitely.

It is very important to understand that acne has several underlying causes and that many treatment options are available. The first step is to recognize the condition. Then, by asking questions and with proper evaluation, we can determine the best treatment plan, which can then be adjusted as necessary based on changing variables such as change of season, hormones, stressors, or other factors.

Acne does not have to be a condition that you accept and try to live with. Much ongoing research on this topic is taking place, and there have been exciting breakthroughs in treatment options, including both topical treatments and oral medications, as well as medical procedures that your dermatologist can provide for you to help guide you back to smooth, even-toned, clear skin as quickly as possible.

I have included the most common questions that I hear in my practice about acne and the answers that I offer to my patients. I have also included many of my patients' personal experiences to help walk you through what you can expect with various aspects of acne and their treatment. My goal is to help you understand that you are not alone in what you are going through and that there is so much that you can do to help yourself. The end result is a better you—from outside and in. Enjoy.

Doris J. Day, MD, MA
July 2004

Dedication

For Kambiz,
Sabrina,
and Andrew
My strength, wisdom and love.

PART ONE

Acne Overview

What is acne?

Who gets acne?

What causes acne?

More . . .

1. What is acne?

The complete medical name for acne is **acne vulgaris**. Vulgaris is Latin for "common," which aptly describes one of the most frequently diagnosed conditions worldwide. Other names that are often used to describe acne are pimples, zits, **lesions**, bumps, breakouts, red spots, clogged pores, **blackheads**, **whiteheads**, and rash. Most people who suffer from acne feel that they are alone in their suffering and that no one has it as bad as they do. The reality is that acne is a very common and often chronic medical condition of the **hair follicles** that line the skin and their associated oil-producing **glands** (see Figure 1). It occurs most commonly on the face, especially in the area known as the "T zone," which includes the forehead, nose, and chin. It can also involve the chest, back, arms, and buttocks.

Certain parts of the body (such as the lips) will never get acne because they have no oil-producing glands. Many factors affect who will get acne, at what age they will get acne, how severely the acne will affect them, and whether they will ever "outgrow" the acne. Ultimately, anyone can get acne at any age—from birth to old age. It is a skin condition that occurs in every gender, race, and ethnicity.

People who were spared acne in their teen years may one day wake up in their 30s or 40s to find a few—or many—pimples. Most commonly, though, acne is a product of teenage years, even if it lasts well beyond those years.

Acne can consist of a single pimple or many lesions. It can look red, or white, or even black. It can be itchy, painful, or merely unsightly. People with either dry skin or oily skin can have acne, although people with

---

Acne vulgaris

The medical name for acne.

Lesion

a mark in the skin.

Blackheads

a type of acne that does not contain active bacteria. The contents of the follicle have turned black after exposure to oxygen.

Whiteheads

a type of acne lesion. White heads are white bumps in the skin that are closed to the surface.

Acne is a very common and often chronic medical condition.

Hair follicles

the unit that contains the hair and the roots of hair.

Glands

a group of cells that make a substance for use in the body.

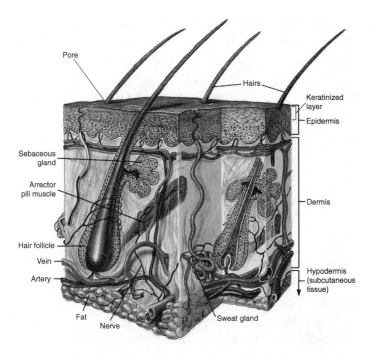

Figure 1. The structure of human skin. (Reproduced from Alters S, *Biology: Understanding Life*. Copyright © 2000 by Jones and Bartlett Publishers, Inc., Sudbury, MA).

oily skin are more prone to acne. Different people may make different types of lesions that can last from days to weeks to months and sometimes leave significant redness or scars.

In all types of acne, the first step in the condition's progression is a combination of increased oil production from the **sebaceous glands** and improper shedding of the skin cells lining the hair follicles. The skin on the face, chest, back, and upper arms all have an increased density of sebaceous glands, which are attached to the hundreds of miniature hairs that exit to the surface of the skin through follicles, commonly called **pores.**

Sebaceous glands

oil-producing glands located in the deeper layers of the skin.

Pores

openings of the follicles to the surface of the skin.

Each follicle has a sebaceous gland attached to it (Figure 2). These glands produce an oily substance called **sebum**, which travels from the sebaceous gland through the follicle and ends on the surface of the skin. At the base of each follicle, a bacterium called *Propionibacterium acnes* (*P. acnes*) is also often present. This bacterium grows and flourishes under certain conditions, such as that of very low or no oxygen concentration. It is the main culprit that is responsible for a certain type of acne called **inflammatory acne**.

Sebum

oil produced by the sebaceous glands.

The upper layer of skin cells that line the follicle normally sloughs off at a regular interval of once every 1 to 2 months; the specific frequency of the sloughing varies depending on the site of the body in which the follicle is located. If the opening of the follicle gets blocked or if the skin cells of the lining regenerate either too quickly or too slowly and do not move up and out of the follicle properly, then problems arise. The next layer of skin cells behind them now have nowhere to go. Additionally, the oxygen supply in the follicle gets cut off, which then allows the *P. acnes* to grow and flourish.

Inflammatory acne

a class of acne where the main lesions are papules, and pustules, not comedones.

The oil that the sebaceous glands produce, called sebum, along with the protein that makes up the skin cells, serves as a perfect diet on which the *P. acnes* grow and prosper and produce more *P. acnes*. At this point the body recognizes that something is amiss and sends its army of **white blood cells** to survey the scene and attack as needed to clear the infection and rid the site of any "foreign" invaders. This leaves the skin looking red and bumpy and, often, feeling itchy or painful.

White blood cells

the body's main defense against infection.

If the *P. acnes* is not activated, then the contents of the follicle build up and bulge behind the blocked opening

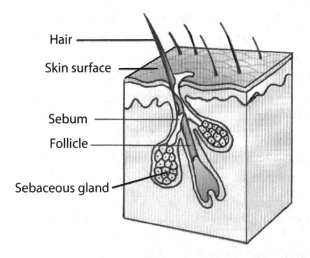

Figure 2. The pilosibaceous unit. (From the National Institute of Musculoskeletal and Skin Diseases, www.niams.nih.gov)

and create a lumpy, bumpy look on the surface of the skin that can be white if the opening remains blocked or black if the contents finally burst through to the surface and react with oxygen. These lesions are called whiteheads and blackheads, respectively. They most commonly occur on the face and back, and seem to be a fixture for most people on their noses.

2. Who gets acne? Do I have acne?

People of all races, ethnicity, and ages get acne, making it the most common skin disorder in the United States. It is most common in adolescents and young adults. Nearly 85% of people between the ages of 12 and 24 years develop the disorder. For some people, acne tends to go away, or at least dramatically improve, by the time they reach their 30s; However, some people in their 40s and 50s continue to suffer from this skin problem, and others do not even start to get acne until they are in their 20s, 30s, 40s, or more.

Genetics

the factors that you inherit from your parents.

Hormone

a chemical substance formed in one organ of the body, such as the adrenal gland, pituitary, or the ovary, etc., that is carried to another organ or tissue where it has a specific effect.

Different people may be prone to different types of acne based on **genetics** and other factors that scientists are still working to understand. Some people may have an increased production of specific **hormones** that trigger acne (see Question 15), whereas others have an increased sensitivity to those hormones. Still others may have specific issues local to the follicles/pores and sebaceous gland that make them more susceptible to acne lesions. Also, some people may be on medications that trigger or worsen acne. Finally, for most, it may be a combination of several of these factors that set off acne flares.

Claudine's comment:

It is difficult enough being a woman executive, surrounded by men, and feeling like I have to prove myself. I have many meetings I have to attend, and I also do a lot of entertaining. Having a breakout of acne really adds to the stress and makes me feel like I just want to hide in my office. I never had acne like this as a teenager, and it is very frustrating to have it now. I get new acne lesions nearly every week, and they seem to last for weeks and weeks, leaving behind red marks that linger for months. I know that stress is a factor for me, but my stress is not going away. My appearance is very important to me, especially with my career, so getting to the bottom of this problem and finding a solution that works has been very important to me.

It is well understood that although acne is a condition specific to the skin, its social and psychologic impact, scarring, and even disfigurement go much deeper. People with acne often think of themselves as socially inferior, unworthy, or socially unacceptable. The same person who exhibits great courage and confidence when his or her skin is clear may shy away from public situations and deny himself or herself many opportunities if he or she has active acne. Even when the acne may seem mild to an outside observer, acne sufferers often isolate themselves and miss out on important opportunities and relationships.

3. How does acne start?

The same skin cells that make up the different layers of the skin also line the hundreds of thousands of follicles that exist within the skin. These follicles with their attached sebaceous glands are most highly concentrated on the face and back. They also exist on the chest, upper arms, and buttocks, but are not as densely concentrated in these areas. The skin cells that line the follicles follow the same pattern as the surrounding skin of migrating toward the surface and sloughing off over time.

For a variety of reasons, not all of which are yet completely understood, acne starts when the sebaceous gland increases production of sebum and the skin cells lining the follicle do not shed properly. Over time, they pile up and block the opening of the follicle. This forms the basic acne lesion, called the **microcomedo**, which is simply an enlarged and plugged hair follicle. This plug is the first step in the formation of any type of acne lesion that follows. The plug is so small that it is invisible, which is why it is called a microcomedo. What happens to this microcomedo determines the type of acne that follows.

Different processes can affect the contents of the follicle, which translates to what happens to the microcomedo and the type of acne that then forms. If the plugged follicle, or microcomedo, stays beneath the

Microcomedo
the first stage of any type of acne lesion. It is so tiny as to be invisible.

skin and continues to grow, it is called a **closed comedo**, which looks like a white bump and thus is called a whitehead. No active bacteria are in a whitehead. The contents are merely the accumulated skin cells and oils that cannot reach the surface because of the blockage from above.

Over time—meaning even a matter of days—the blockage sometimes reaches the surface of the skin and opens. The lesion is then called a blackhead because it looks black on the skin's surface. This black discoloration is not due to dirt. It is due to a process called **oxidation**, in which air and the oils and proteins in the skin all affect each other and cause the contents in the follicle to turn black. Because this mixture is so thick in comparison to the normal contents of the skin, the contents remain in the follicle and continue to block the follicular opening. As with the whitehead, no active bacteria exist in a blackhead. Both whiteheads and blackheads may stay stuck in the skin for a long time.

These lesions are best treated with gentle **exfoliation** and **retinoids** (see Question 7). Surgical extraction can be very effective; however, it is important to remember that fingernails are not surgical instruments and that picking at these lesions, no matter how tempting it is, can make them worse and can increase the risk of scarring (see Questions 12 and 13).

4. What does acne look like?

All acne lesions start as a microcomedo. This consists of a microscopic plug of the follicle. The different types of acne lesions that evolve from the microcomedo are named based on what they look like and whether there are active *P. acnes* at work causing a

Closed comedo

a type of acne lesion that looks white. There is no active bacteria in this type of lesion.

Oxidation

changes that occur after exposure to oxygen.

Exfoliation

the process of removing the upper layers of dead skin.

Retinoids

products, generally in the vitamin A family, that act at specific sites called retinoic acid receptors.

Picking at these lesions, no matter how tempting it is, can make them worse.

localized infection. Since the microcomedo is the earliest step in the process of acne, but is not visible from the surface of the skin, it becomes important to treat acne-prone skin regularly and completely before pimples even appear visible to the eyes, in order to minimize scarring and to clear lesions that do appear as quickly as possible. Once the acne lesions become visible, they can be white or black, as described above, or red. They can be as small as a pinpoint or over 1 inch in size. They can be in the upper layers of the skin or deeper within the skin. They can last from days to weeks to months and can resolve with little or no consequence, or they can leave behind changes in skin color and texture that can be quite disconcerting.

The main types of lesions that we see in acne have traditionally been divided into two types, noninflammatory and inflammatory, as follows:

1. Noninflammatory (no active *P. acnes*, see Figure 3)
   • **Whiteheads**: The plugged follicle that stays beneath the skin and continues to grow is called a closed comedo in medical lingo—or more commonly a whitehead because it looks like a white bump just under the skin. The problem is that there is a very natural inclination to try to pick the white core, which then leads to redness and local infection because the fingers used to pick at the lesion are never sterile; this in turn leads to an increased risk of infection and scarring. It is now known that there is in fact some inflammation associated with this type of lesion so the term non-inflammatory is somewhat of a misnomer. The significance of such findings is that treatments initially thought to be appropriate only for

9

inflammatory types of lesions are now also used very effectively in the treatment of non-inflammatory types of acne.

- **Blackheads**: A comedo that reaches the surface of the skin and opens is called a blackhead because it looks black on the skin's surface. This black discoloration is not due to dirt. Both whiteheads and blackheads may stay in the skin for a long time. The temptation is to pick out the black core, but again, as is true of picking at any type of acne lesion, this can lead to redness and scarring. It is now known that there is in fact inflammation associated with this type of lesion as well. The significance of these findings is that treatments initially thought to be appropriate only for inflammatory types of lesions are now also used very effectively in the treatment of non-inflammatory types of acne.

2. Inflammatory (contains active *P. acnes* within the follicle)

- **Papules**: These are inflamed (red, swollen) lesions that usually appear as small, pink bumps on the skin and can be itchy or tender to the touch.
- **Pustules**: These are papules that are topped with pus and may be red at the base. The pus consists of dead white blood cells and bacteria that are a result of a "war" between the white blood cells and the *P. acnes* in the follicle that then overflowed to the surface of the skin.
- **Nodules**: These are large, painful, solid, or fluctuant lesions that are lodged deep within the skin with a small opening to the surface where the follicle exits to the skin. They often feel hard to

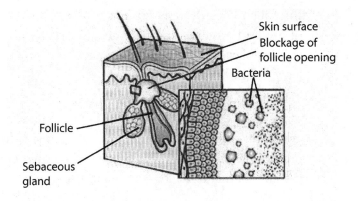

Skin surface
Blockage of
follicle opening
Bacteria

Follicle

Sebaceous
gland

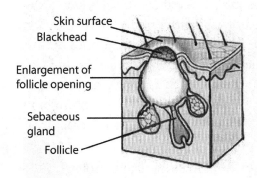

Skin surface
Blackhead

Enlargement of
follicle opening

Sebaceous
gland
Follicle

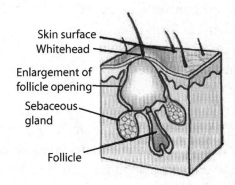

Skin surface
Whitehead

Enlargement of
follicle opening

Sebaceous
gland

Follicle

**Figure 3. Noninflammatory acne. (From the National Institute of Muscu-
loskeletal and Skin Diseases, www.niams.nih.gov)**

the touch because they consist of a combination of oils and proteins that have accumulated within the nodular cavity. They can last for months and leave behind crater-like scars.

- **Cysts**: These are rarely found in acne, and the term is generally abandoned in favor of nodulo-cystic or severe nodular acne. This consists of multiple deep, painful, pus-filled lesions that can leave behind crater-like scarring in the skin.

The acne lesions may be localized to only one area or may cover several areas of the body. They may occur on only the face in some people, or on only the back or chest. In others, they occur on only the buttocks, whereas in still others it occurs at several sites at one time. There can be any given type of lesion or combination of types of lesions at any given area at any time. Having one type of acne lesion does not exclude you from having other types of acne lesions at the same time.

There is something about an acne infection with active *P. acnes* that makes the body react differently than it does to other types of infection from other organisms. For some reason the body breaks down *P. acnes* much more slowly than it breaks down other invaders. Also, to make matters worse, the immune response magnifies the inflammatory process even more. The combination of these two factors means that lesions take a long time to clear up, and that the lesions themselves appear red and irritated. On top of this, picking at an acne pimple makes the inflammation worse, even if the acne is otherwise being treated properly. If you pop an acne pimple, the redness often lingers for a very long time, which means that the skin stays red and irritated looking for even longer.

The treatments recommended to you will depend on the types of lesions you have, how often you break out, whether you scar from the acne, and how many body areas are involved. Many of the treatment options overlap and address various types of acne lesions, which makes it easier to determine an effective treatment plan.

5. What causes acne?

We know much about more about acne than we used to. We know what it looks like. We know a lot of different ways to treat it, and we know that it can be a chronic and more than annoying condition that can last, on and off, for years. What we still do not know is the exact cause of acne. This is one reason that there is still no actual cure for acne. The current school of thought is that acne results from several, if not many, related factors.

There is still no actual cure for acne.

Whatever the causes of acne in terms of internal or external factors, acne is, in the end, a condition of the skin with well-defined players such as skin cells, sebaceous glands, and follicles (pores), along with *P. acnes* bacteria that live at the base of the pore (Table 1).

In any given individual, acne can be a generalized process involving many areas of the body or a very localized process involving only the nose or the forehead or the area around the mouth. It can sometimes occur only on the back, sparing the face entirely. Even when localized to only one relatively small body area, it can be persistent, scarring, and very difficult to control.

When looking at the underlying cause of acne, two general categories need to be considered: One is the

Acne Overview

Table 1. Factors Involved in Causing Acne

Factor	Description
Inflammatory cells	Trigger response to infection
Keratinocytes	Skin cells
Pilosebaceous unit	Sebaceous gland with attached hair follicle
Sebaceous glands	Oil-producing glands
P. acnes	Bacteria specific to the follicles in the skin
Androgens	Types of hormones important in acne

intrinsic nature of the person—his or her genetic and hormonal makeup, the sensitivity of follicles to specific hormones, and local environment. The second category is the extrinsic circumstances. This is a much larger and more varied category over which we have more control. It can also be divided into internal factors, such as medications and internal stressors, and external (extrinsic) factors, such as external stressors and products used on the skin (Table 2). Recent studies have shown that some of the changes that lead to the inflammatory types of acne occur behind the scenes in what otherwise looks like perfectly normal skin. This means that the underlying causes of acne can sometimes be addressed even before the acne becomes obvious on the surface of the skin.

This has led to a revolutionary change in the way doctors recommend **topical** treatments for acne. In the past, "spot" treatment, meaning treating only the pimples themselves, was the norm for many of the medicines commonly recommended; however, the new recommendation is changing to one in which the

Topical

a product that is used on the skin, such as a cream, lotion, or gel.

Table 2.   Acne Instigators

Intrinsic (related to genetics or factors that are out of your direct control)
- Family history of severe acne
- Increased circulating androgens
- Hyperresponsiveness of follicles to androgens
- Local abnormalities of the pilosebaceous unit

Extrinsic (related to factors that you have at least some control over)
- Internal
  - Medications
  - Stress
  - Oral contraceptives
  - Other hormonal treatments
- External
  - Makeup
  - Pollution
  - Occlusive products
  - Irritants

entire area should be targeted, even if the skin appears normal on the surface, because the acne may be brewing underneath. Also, some areas should be treated **prophylactically** (preventatively) in order to avoid the acne from occurring in the first place.

Hormonal changes related to pregnancy or starting or stopping birth control pills can improve acne in some women but cause acne or make it worse in people already prone to acne, depending on the **oral contraceptive** used (see Questions 79–81). Our bodies are constantly fine tuning themselves both internally and externally to adjust to change within our bodies and from the world around us. Something is always going on.

Changes in sleep cycles, exams, foods, relationships, and experiences—both good and bad—all affect our bodies on different levels. Internally, this means that there are constant small but significant shifts in various

Acne Overview

Prophylactically

a treatment or medication in the absence of active disease, in order to prevent the condition from recurring.

Oral contraceptive

medications used by women to help prevent unwanted pregnancy.

15

hormones to cope with these changes that affect our moods, **metabolism,** and skin.

Metabolism

our bodies' natural energy requirements.

From the outside, the situations that can bring out the acne or make it worse can be from the certain products that we apply to our skin, using our fingers to pick at the skin, the effects of pollution, wind, sun, and other factors that may eventually get translated into acne or irritation that can look like acne.

It is the combination of internal and external events that throws our skin off balance and can aggravate acne. For example, some of the products that are applied to the skin get concentrated around the pores, which means that a higher concentration of the product ends up being in that area. This can often trigger a process in the skin that sometimes looks exactly like the inflammatory types of acne but is really just an irritant reaction in the skin.

The temptation here is to treat the condition as if it were acne, only to worsen the condition. The lesson here is that if your treatment is not working within a reasonable period of time, which I consider to be 2 to 4 weeks, it is time to see your dermatologist and get professional advice. To avoid such a situation, it is also important that you write down all your questions before a doctor visit and bring a list of the products that you are using or have used in the past so that you can review with your doctor which may be appropriate or which you should avoid.

6. What specific role does the sebaceous gland play?

Acne occurs in areas where there is the highest density of active sebaceous glands. It is usually found on the face, back, chest, and upper arms, occasionally extending to the buttocks in some cases. The sebaceous gland

Table 3. Sebaceous Lipid Composition

Triglycerides	56%
Wax esters	26%
Squalene	15%
Cholesterol	2%
Cholesterol esters	1%

is important in the context of its effects on the **pilose-baceous unit**, which is the grouping of the sebaceous gland and its attached hair follicle.

The major product of sebaceous glands is sebum, which is a type of lipid (fat) (Table 3). Some of the triglycerides in sebum are converted to free fatty acids by *P. acnes*, which further creates an environment in which the *P. acnes* can comfortably grow and flourish. **Squalene** and certain free fatty acids play an important role in the causation of acne. It is also known that the sebum of people with acne has relatively little linoleic acid. This is a type of free fatty acid that the skin requires to help turnover and slough off properly.

In animal models where there is not enough linoleic acid, the skin becomes scaly. You can think of the acne lesion as one large scale existing inside the follicle. As a group, people with acne have larger sebaceous glands and produce more sebum, which may dilute the linoleic acid in the follicle and in this way disrupt normal skin sloughing and help produce the microcomedo.

Excessive sebum production is the first abnormality that occurs in the onset of acne and is usually followed by abnormal sloughing of the skin cells lining

Pilosebaceous unit
the grouping containing the hair follicle and attached sebaceous gland.

Squalene
found in the sebum, squalene is an important precursor to androgen production.

Acne Overview

17

Comedogenic

products that induce open or closed comedones to form after about 2 to 3 weeks of use.

Androgens

a class of hormones including testosterone and DHEAS. They cause the sebaceous gland to enlarge and produce more sebum, which is an important factor in the causation of acne.

Puberty

age at which certain hormones, called sex hormones, kick in followed by specific changes, such as menses in girls and beard growth in boys.

Heredity

the traits you get from your parents, such as tendency to acne, hair color, height, etc.

Acne needs to be addressed from several different angles.

the pores, leading to the microcomedo. Sebum is known to be **comedogenic**. Also, in studies in which sebum was injected into the skin, the result was inflammation, making sebum both an inflammatory substance and comedogenic.

In people who are prone to acne, starting when they are approximately 7 to 8 years old, the overall size of the sebaceous gland increases and becomes lumpier in response to increased production of hormones called **androgens**. This process is accompanied by increased secretion of sebaceous oils, called sebum. The hormonal changes at **puberty** that follow lead to changes in both the sebaceous glands and the skin cells lining the hair follicle opening (pore). Also, there are factors that control how the sebaceous gland handles the hormone, which is why some people are more affected by hormones than others. This is where **heredity** plays a role. In acne, excess sebum production is mainly due to differences in the response of the pilosebaceous unit to the local environment, increased circulating androgens, or both. This is why acne needs to be addressed from several different angles, even if there is no measurable hormonal imbalance. It is also why women with no measurable abnormalities in hormone levels often find that their acne improves when they take oral contraceptives for other reasons.

7. Why do my pores keep getting bigger? What can I do about it?

Pore size is one of the top concerns patients have when they come in for a visit. We know that pores are the openings of the follicles to the surface of the skin. They are supposed to be there. Everyone has them. They are more obvious in some people than in others;

however, "my pores are bigger than anyone else I know" is a common complaint.

We know that there is a lot going on in those follicles, and we know that there are many influences affecting the contents and size. The problem is that pores are always too big when they are on your face, as opposed to someone else's, and there does not seem to be anything great available to help you get rid of them.

Amy's comments:

I know I stare at my face a lot, but I am really concerned that my pores keep getting bigger and bigger. They are out of control. I have tried facials and over-the-counter treatments, but nothing helps. I check my face out every morning and night in my special magnification mirror. It helps me see all the flaws in my skin. Every time I look, the first things I see are my humongous pores. I feel like the pores are taking over my face.

The first thing that I recommend is to get rid of the magnified mirror if you are using one to study your pores. Even though you will never believe it, no one sees your pores the way you do. I have never had a conversation with someone and heard him or her say this: "Did you see how big their pores were?" It has never happened. We notice a lot of things about other people and about ourselves. "Really big pores" seems like something that most people see only in themselves.

Get rid of the magnified mirror if you are using one to study your pores.

Genetics, sun exposure, and hormones affect pore size. Pores appear larger and more prominent with increased age. Treatments are available that can, at least temporarily, help minimize the appearance of pores. Regular exfoliation, along with the use of a class of topical treatments called retinoids, can help skin cells turnover/regenerate more normally and can control the activity of the sebaceous glands that contribute to the enlarged appearance of the pores.

Amy's comments:

I started a strict sun protection regimen, and I also now regularly use Retin-A on my whole face. This has helped, but it took me a while to get used to using the Retin-A. I started by using the Retin-A every day, even though I was warned this might irritate my skin. I just thought that since my skin feels so oily, I would be able to tolerate it. Well, I couldn't. At first my skin got very red. It felt like I had a sunburn. I stopped using the Retin-A for a few days, and my doctor gave me a prescription for a topical cortisone cream to use for 1 week. When my skin calmed down, I started the Retin-A again, this time more slowly, and I did just fine. Now I try not to stare at my face all the time, and I use a cover powder that really helps too. I started to get lots of compliments on my skin, and that was a real boost.

In the end, there are some things you can do to help your pores appear smaller. Always start with sun protection. This is the easiest way to eliminate one factor that leads to increased pore size. Aside from that, several different treatments are available that have some effect on pore size, mostly as a temporary or secondary effect. From the least invasive/intense end of the treatment/concealing spectrum, it is important to note that a huge number of cosmetic companies have invested millions in making and marketing powders, creams, and lotions that will help to conceal your pores. This is the simplest way to manage the problem, but it clearly does not "solve" it. No true solution exists because pores are a natural part of the skin, so looking for appropriate powders and creams that can camouflage the pores can be very useful.

A good place to start along the topical treatment spectrum are retinoids, since they do affect sebaceous gland activity and can improve the appearance of pores; however, this treatment can be drying or irritating to the skin and is not for everyone. **Facials** can help temporarily; however, the pores refill relatively quickly, and if the facials are not done well, they can lead to irritation of the skin (see Question 37).

Next down the line are the **lasers** and **intense pulsed light treatments** (see Question 89). These are considered cosmetic treatments that, over time, help to decrease the appearance of pores. Multiple treatments are usually necessary, and the results can vary from person to person. Although there is no permanent way available today to eliminate pores, I believe that the laser and intense pulsed light technology come closest to offering long-lasting, safe results over time.

At the most extreme end of the treatment spectrum are medications such as oral isotretinoin are known, at least temporarily, to decrease sebaceous gland activity. This would most certainly not be a first-line treatment for enlarged pores without the presence of severe, scarring acne; however, it is one of the benefits of the therapy.

8. What are the different types of acne?

There are several subtypes of acne. Identifying the different types is important because they often have different underlying causes that can be specifically addressed and because sometimes different treatments

Facial

various skin treatments, usually done by an aesthetician, with the intention of improving the skin.

Lasers

machines that produce single bands of light, with different lasers being able to produce different single bands. These bands can be used to target various elements in the skin to help improve skin texture, tone, and quality and to treat acne.

Intense pulsed light treatments

treatments using a broad band of visible and near infrared wavelengths of light that block out other wavelengths. This produces broad bands of light that can penetrate various depths of skin and target both red and brown lesions, and can treat acne.

Table 4. Types of Acne

Acne vulgaris	the most common type of acne consisting of papules, pustules, and comedones in various combinations. There are several subtypes:
Comedonal acne	mostly blackheads and whiteheads
Inflammatory acne	mostly papules, pustules, cysts
Nodular acne	scattered nodules mostly concentrated on the face, chest, and/or back
Cystic acne	scattered cystic lesions in common acne areas
Neonatal acne	an acne-like eruption that can occur in newborns or infants.
Acne excoriée	even mild acne may be severely disfiguring when accompanied by extensive excoriations (picking) at lesions.
Pomade acne	caused by occlusive hair products.
Acne cosmetica	caused by occlusive makeup and skin-care products.
Steroid acne	results from long-term use of oral or topical steroids.
Acne conglobata	an unusually severe form of cystic acne that consists of large abscesses with interconnecting sinuses, cysts, and grouped inflammatory nodules.
Acne keloidalis	a type of acne in which healing results in keloidal scarring. This is most common at the nape of the neck but also occurs on the arms, chest, and back. It is unusual to see keloids on the face, although they can occur at the jaw line and under the chin and can sometimes grow to be very itchy, painful, and disfiguring.

are required for best results (Table 4). These different types can occur in various combinations in any given individual and can look similar. It can be very helpful to classify the type of acne that you have in terms of treatment, evaluation of risk of scarring, and prevention of future breakouts.

9. What is neonatal acne?

Acne in newborns (neonatal acne) is one of the more common eruptions, occurring in approximately 20% of newborns. It typically appears at approximately 2 to 3 weeks of life and looks like small, red bumps and pustules that are scattered over the cheeks of the newborn child. The forehead, eyelids, chin, neck, and upper chest may also become involved.

Acne or acne-like breakouts in newborns can be difficult to diagnose accurately because there are different, usually temporary and harmless conditions of the skin that often look very similar but have different underlying causes. Several temporary hormonal imbalances can occur in the neonatal period that may play a role in the newborn period; however, comedones, which are the typical lesion seen on adolescent acne, are not seen in acne of the newborn. There can also be involvement of a yeast called *Pityrosporum* rather than *P. acnes* or the conditions that normally cause acne. This type of rash is not harmful to the child and can be treated with a topical antifungal that the baby's doctor prescribes.

Controversy exists regarding the true nature of neonatal acne, some arguing that it is not truly acne but a rash that looks like acne with different underlying causes, but because the condition most commonly resolves on its own, the discussion is mostly academic. When treatment is offered, it is usually in the form of a combination of antifungal creams along with a variety of creams typically used in the treatment of acne. Sometimes oral medications are used if warranted.

Infantile acne presents as comedones and inflammatory lesions, similar to the way adolescent acne would look. It can occur at anywhere from 2 months to 2 years of age or more. Baby boys are more commonly affected than girls. The face is typically involved. The underlying cause is thought to be hormonal.

This type of acne is relatively uncommon, and in these cases, there is sometimes a family history of severe, scarring acne. Once diagnosed, the acne is usually treated with appropriate oral or topical **antibiotics** in conjunction with topical **benzoyl peroxide** (BP) and low concentration of **tretinoin** (Retin-A). Unlike with neonatal acne, early treatment is important in even mild cases, as there is a significant risk of scarring. **Tetracyclines** are not used in this age group.

10. At what age do adolescents (teens) start to get acne?

Girls typically start to get acne when their hormones kick in (approximately 11 to 13 years old), which is about the time that they start their period. Boys start to get acne at the age of approximately 12 years, with a range of 9 to 15 years old. As most girls will attest, boys on average mature later than girls.

Jonathan's comments:

I can't believe this is happening to me. I am now 14 years old. I like to think of myself as a good-looking guy, and I am pretty popular at school. Now I feel like I am about to lose everything. My face looks absolutely horrible. I have red bumps all over my face, and I spend hours getting rid of these bumps that are deep under my skin. The problem is that I then get a swollen red bump that is huge and that won't go away for weeks or months. I keep getting new ones, especially around tests, and my social life and self-esteem are really starting to suffer. I don't want to approach girls, and I try not to go out unless I have to.

Antibiotics

a large category of drugs that target bacteria.

Benzoyl peroxide (BP)

an antiseptic commonly used topically in the treatment of acne. It does not induce bacterial resistance.

Tretinoin (Retin-A)

medication commonly used in the treatment of acne vulgaris. This compound is in the vitamin A family.

Tetracyclines

class of antibiotics typically used in the treatment of acne vulgaris.

Early on in the onset of teen acne, the main lesions are blackheads and whiteheads. Later in puberty, there is a higher incidence of inflammatory lesions. Early lesions usually occur around the center of the face and on the forehead. Teenagers are usually active and have very busy school and after-school schedules as well as increasingly active social lives. Being a teenager is tough enough as it is without adding the complicating factor of acne. Unfortunately, one pimple can make the difference between popularity and outcast in the mind of many teens.

This means that treatment for teenagers must be simple, efficient, and (ideally) must travel well in order to encourage compliance. Results must also come relatively quickly for this age group, more than any other, because self-esteem often rides on the latest zit that has come or gone. Combinations of oral and topical treatments work very well in these young adults. It is also very important for parents and dermatologists to have a good dialogue in order to promote better understanding of the teenager's skin condition.

Some parents are more upset about the acne than their children, whereas others feel their children are overreacting and that acne does not need to be treated at all because it is just a "cosmetic" problem. Other parents may believe that acne is simply an age-related rite of passage that does not need to be addressed because their child will eventually "outgrow" it. After all, acne is only a passing condition of the skin, right? Now you know that this is most certainly wrong. Acne can be a very serious disfiguring condition that the teen may or may not outgrow. Many wonderful treatments can help to control the acne and prevent scarring and other problems. Doctors can make a big difference by improving communication between parents and teens.

Jonathan's comments:

It took a while to see results, but I finally am getting back into my old life. I have a few scars from areas that I picked, but I am more careful now. I do still panic a little when I see a new zit; however, I have medicine to put on it, and my doctor gives me an injection of cortisone right into the pimple if I need. I have these cool travel packs that I keep in by backpack at all times to sop up all the oil that accumulates on my skin during the day. My new girlfriend is into all of these skin care products, and she got me a face scrub that smells really cool. I still have my bad days, but now I look at my friends and am starting to see them go through the same thing. I try to tell them it's no big deal, but they just don't get it. I don't know why they are such babies about it.

Teens need special attention and counseling in order to maximize the benefits of treatment. Because teenagers are minors, parents also need to be educated and encouraged to take their teenager's acne very seriously. There are several reasons to treat acne in teens and to take it very seriously, as outlined here. The social stigma of acne and the risk of scarring, which is generally permanent, are the two biggest reasons. The availability of wonderful, easy-to-use treatments that are safe and effective makes acne one of the relatively easier teen "conditions" to address and offers a compelling reason why the condition must not be ignored.

11. What is pomade acne?

Pomade acne

a type of acne due to ingredients used in the hair.

Pomade acne was first reported in 1970 in African-American men who used scalp creams and oils regularly. It consisted of blackheads and whiteheads (mostly on the temple and forehead). In the original studies, several products were implicated in the acne, including products that contained mineral oil and Vaseline or other petrolatum-based ingredients, among other ingredients. It is thought that the occlusive nature of the pomades was at least partially to blame. Patients with pomade acne are often advised to use hair care products that are noncomedogenic or less comedogenic, such as products that are water or **glycerin** based.

It is important to understand that no matter what you put in your hair, by the end of the day, some of it will end up on your face. Pomade acne is now a more common problem (seen in all skin types) because hair products and styles have become more complicated and often intricate, requiring pomades to keep the hair in place.

It is very important to evaluate the products that you are using in your hair if you are finding that the distribution of your acne is more concentrated at the edges of your face and if you have longer hair that sits against the sides of your neck. Once the offending product is discontinued, the acne will eventually clear up on its own but can very effectively be treated with topical anti-acne therapy to expedite the resolution of the acne and to minimize any scarring.

12. How long should a typical pimple last?

Some people note that their pimples last for months before finally going away. Comedones can last for weeks or months or longer if not treated. Inflammatory lesions usually clear within days to weeks; however, marks (red and eventually brown) can be left behind that remain for months longer. Also, because

Glycerin

a common additive in soaps and moisturizers to increase the moisture content of the skin.

Acne Overview

acne can recur in the same spot—sometimes just as the lesion is beginning to clear—it can flare again, which makes it seem like it is lasting for months.

Cysts tend to be recurrent in the same spot, and you may notice that they increase and decrease in size over time, seemingly on their own. The temptation, as usual, is to pick at these lesions to get rid of them, but this only aggravates them and usually makes them last longer. It also increases the risk of scarring.

One of the worst things that you can do to a pimple of any type is to pick or squeeze it. The trauma and irritation caused from the picking or squeezing may give you an immediate feeling of satisfaction that you have cleared the contents and made the skin smoother; however, in the short run, it makes the area redder and more prone to having a brown mark or depressed scar left behind, and worst of all, it doesn't stop the pimple from coming back in the same place next time.

The main goal for an acne sufferer is to try to prevent the pimple from forming in the first place. Once it does come up, the first trick for getting an acne lesion to clear more quickly and to be less likely to resolve without scarring is to avoid picking at it; second, treat it early with an appropriate antibacterial/anti-inflammatory medication. Finally, minimize putting anything on it or doing anything to it that will excessively irritate the pimples. It also helps to evaluate any causes that you think might be behind the breakout. Was it around an exam or a particularly stressful project? Did you use any new creams or lotions? Did you start or stop any medications or oral contraceptives? Could anything else have contributed? Finally, if the lesion does not go away, it is a good idea to have the spot evaluated by your dermatologist to make sure that it is simply a pimple that is slow to heal and not something else that would be addressed differently.

13. Sometimes I feel like there is something under my skin (in the pimple) and that I need to get it out. Is picking at my pimples really bad for my skin?

There is a name for the type of acne that occurs from constant picking at or squeezing the lesions. It is called **acne excoriée**. A number of people feel that their skin must always feel smooth at any cost. They feel that if they could just get the contents of the pimple out, the pimple will go away and the skin will heal. Even though they see that the result is scarring and that picking does not solve the problem, the picking continues and perpetuates the acne. Actually, even as the skin heals, there can be a feeling that something hard is under the skin, and the temptation is, again, to pick it.

Acne excoriée
the medical name for acne that has been picked at or scratched repeatedly.

Caryn's comments:

I have a 5× magnifying mirror in my bathroom that helps me see every little spot on my skin. I stare at my pores. They look huge, and the pimples are absolutely unsightly. I can feel that there is something in them, and I know for a fact that until I get that hard substance out, the pimple or bump will not go away. The bumps seem to last forever, and the only way I can move things along is by getting that stuff out from under my skin.

Several processes occur in acne. The first is the part that causes the acne, and second is the part that heals

Follicular plug

blockage of the opening of the follicles. This is the one of the first steps in all types of acne.

the acne. In active acne, there is the **follicular plug**, the comedo, and some degree of inflammation. This can feel hard and can last for days to even weeks. The healing part also takes time will often feel like there is a bump or somewhat hard substance under the skin which can last from weeks to months.

The problem is that picking makes matters only worse. No matter how much you wash your hands, bacteria still exists on your hands and under your nails and will transfer to your facial skin. Also, there is no way that you can be accurate enough in focusing on only the acne lesion without irritating the surrounding skin to some extent. This picked skin then has to heal itself and can again feel like there is a hard substance under the skin from the scab that forms, or from the scarring process within the skin that is trying to recover.

Caryn's comments:

When I pick at my skin, I always wash my hands first; I then try to squeeze around the bump to get the stuff out. If that doesn't work I try to make the opening bigger using either my nail or the tip of a pin that I have wiped with an alcohol swab. Sometimes it bleeds, and sometimes I can get out what looks like a little white ball of gunk. The problem is that it then takes forever for the redness to go away, and the stuff inside just seems to come back again. I end up with marks all over my face, and then I don't want to go out or be seen. I know I should just let it run its course, but I am convinced that if I can just get that stuff out from under the skin, it would all go away. Then I just have to treat the scars.

One of the worst consequences of acne is the scarring.

Undoubtedly one of the worst consequences of acne is the scarring that is left behind. Unfortunately, the chances of scarring are only increased when lesions are picked at. The solution is to treat the acne with appropriate medications and to avoid touching the lesions at any cost. Your dermatologist can extract the contents of the pimples for you, or inject the lesions with a dilute solution of cortisone to help individual lesions resolve more quickly. In time, as the lesions heal and fewer new pimples occur, the skin will feel naturally smoother and will look healthier as well.

14. Why does my face feel greasier throughout the day?

Sebum production is lowest at night and increases throughout the day. Since the highest concentration of sebaceous glands is on the face, especially in the "T zone," this increased production of sebum during the day can make your face feel greasier. Sebaceous gland activity also increases in response to hormones, stressors, and irritants. The face can also feel greasier throughout the day depending on products used on the face and in the hair. The heavier the product, the more likely it is to be occlusive and cause buildup of sebum on the skin. There are also sweat glands on the skin, and in times of increased heat or stress, these glands increase production of sweat which, when combined with sebum, makes the skin look shinier and feel oilier.

For women, increased sebum production begins approximately 1 week before the **menstrual period**, which also makes the face feel oilier. It can be very helpful to carry blotting pads that are specifically designed to absorb this oily mixture off the skin and thus provide at least temporary relief. It can also be

Menstrual period
the monthly, cyclical bleeding cycle women experience when they are not pregnant. Irregularities in this cycle can indicate hormonal imbalance that can be an aggravating factor in acne.

helpful to address the underlying issue by controlling body temperature as much as possible, managing stressors, and using products that help minimize sebum production when possible. These would include products that contain **salicylic acid** or **retinols**.

Salicylic acid

ingredient that helps exfoliate the upper layers of the skin. It is commonly found in over the counter acne treatment products.

Retinol

vitamin A.

15. What role do hormones play?

Hormones are everywhere in the body. They are constantly released into the blood to help the body adjust to increased activity, internal and external stressors, incoming food that needs to be digested, and stress, stress, and more stress... and did I already mention stress? It is incredible how such a small amount of a substance can have such far-reaching and profound effects on so many different organ systems.

Hormones, specifically androgens or sex hormones, also play a critical role in acne on many levels. Simply put, if there are no androgens, there is no acne. However, androgens alone are not the sole cause of acne since, as we've seen, many other factors are also involved such as bacterial overgrowth, the manner in which skin cells differentiate and the stickiness of the skin cells. Most standard acne therapies address these components of acne rather than the hormonal component. Severe acne can be a clue to a potentially serious underlying hormonally influenced condition in women called **polycystic ovary syndrome**, which carries certain risks and should be diagnosed and treated appropriately both in terms of general health issues and for better results in treating the acne. One important factor in the cause of acne is an increase in hormones called stress hormones and another called androgens (sex hormones) (Table 5).

Polycystic ovary syndrome

a hormonal condition in women where the ovaries overproduce specific hormones. This can be manifest in the skin as increased and more severe acne, increased hair growth on the face, and hair loss on the scalp.

Table 5. Hormones in Acne

Androgens
DHEAS
Testosterone
17-Hydroxyprogesterone

Stress Hormones
Cortisol

Specific hormone levels increase in both boys and girls during puberty and cause the sebaceous glands to enlarge and increase production of sebum. As we have seen, the types of hormones that lead to acne and that can make acne worse are called androgens, which appear during puberty in greater quantities. Increased sebum production because of androgens acting at the sebaceous follicle is always a prerequisite for acne even after the teenage years. This is why acne is generally worse in areas where there is a higher density of sebaceous glands, such as the face and upper back, and generally absent in areas where you don't have any sebaceous glands such as the elbows and the feet.

There are two ways that these hormones affect acne. In some people, too much hormone is circulating in the blood, therefore triggering acne. In most acne patients, however, there are normal blood levels of androgens, while there is an increased and inappropriate responsiveness of the pilosebaceous unit to a normal amount of circulating androgen. This means that even though all the blood tests come back normal, your body, at the level of the sebaceous gland, is overly accepting of the androgens that are circulating in the blood. The end result is acne.

I often use the analogy of ships coming into port. The ships are the cells carrying the androgen, and the port is the pilosebaceous unit. Usually a ship will come into port, dock, unload its goods, and move on. When the port is full, it will not allow any more ships to dock and unload their goods. In some cases, the port keeps accepting more ships anyway and does not let a ship go by without accepting the goods. This leads to a dock overloaded with goods. In the skin, this situation results in a hormonal pattern of acne. Sometimes there is a combination of both too much androgen circulating in the blood and an overly accepting sebaceous gland in the skin.

Adrenal glands
small, hormone-producing organs that are found near the kidneys.

Before the onset of puberty, between the ages of 7 and 8 years, the **adrenal glands** of both boys and girls produce increasing amounts of types of androgen called dehydroepiandrosterone sulfate (DHEAS) and testosterone, which in turn can be metabolized to more potent androgens in the skin that cause the sebaceous gland to enlarge and increase sebum production. As girls mature, the ovaries take over this role from the adrenal glands, for the most part. The serum level of DHEAS correlates with the severity of comedonal acne in prepubertal girls. In addition, acne severity increases with sexual maturity in both boys and girls, thus with the increased presence of androgens in the body. Therefore, hormonal influences clearly have an important role in the pathogenesis of acne.

Both boys and girls may have acne that is related to increased sensitivity of the sebaceous gland to androgens. In girls, excess ovarian and adrenal production of androgens may also cause acne, particularly when it occurs in older girls/women, is persistent, or is associated with increased hair growth on the face. In girls with acne caused by high circulating androgen levels, free **testosterone** and DHEAS in particular may be present. Low levels of a protein called sex hormone-binding globulin may also be observed. Sex hormone binding globulin attaches to testosterone and helps keep it from affecting the skin. A lack of this globulin translates into greater amounts of androgen circulating in the blood and thereby able to affect the skin.

Testosterone
a male sex hormone.

Androgens are not the only hormones that affect acne. When the body is under stress, whether from fear of an approaching perceived physical or emotional danger, it releases a hormone called **cortisol**. This hormone helps us through whatever situation is at hand, but it does so at a price. Cortisol also leads to suppression of the **immune system**, which gives *P. acnes* an opportunity to flourish, leading to a flare of inflammatory acne in some people.

Immune system
the collection of cells and structures in the body that fight disease or infection. White blood cells, lymph nodes, and lymph vessels are the primary components of the immune system.

In women with insulin resistance associated with increased androgens, improvement in the blood levels of androgens has been observed when medications that improve insulin sensitivity are given. It remains to be seen whether this has a significant effect on improving the acne as well.

16. Is acne contagious?

The bacterium *P. acnes* plays an important role in the inflammatory types of acne; however, it lives in the depths of the hair follicle where it is not easily accessible, even by close contact. This bacterium is not typically active except under certain conditions of

35

very low oxygen concentration such as when the opening of the pore is blocked off from the surface of the skin, which cuts off the oxygen supply. This makes the chances of spreading the bacterium even less likely because there is less access to the outside world.

By the time you see a pustule, it means that your body has reacted to the infection and the pus is mostly a mixture of a lot of dead bacteria, white blood cells, and skin cells, along with other very complicated but minute factors that create inflammation.

P. acnes can also colonize the nose, where it can then be responsible for local spread of acne to the face and back through contact, such as from touching the nose and then touching the face or back. However, acne is not known to spread from person to person and is not considered contagious.

Acne is not known to spread from person to person.

17. What role does heredity play?

Another important factor in both the age of onset of acne and the possible severity and risk of scarring from acne is heredity, or genetics. Researchers believe that the tendency to develop acne, especially severe acne, can be inherited from your parents. For example, studies have shown that many school-age boys with acne have a family history of the condition.

This does not mean that if one or both of your parents had acne that you are necessarily destined to have acne yourself. However, it does indicate that you have a higher chance of getting acne than someone without a family history of acne. It also means that if you do develop acne, it should be treated early in its onset before any scarring or long-term effects occur. In families with strong histories of severe acne, it is very helpful to let your dermatologist know the family history and consider very close and regular follow-up of the acne. In these cases, early evaluation and early treatment mean that severe scarring acne can be diagnosed earlier and that the sometimes disfiguring scars can be avoided or at least greatly minimized.

18. What are the factors that can make acne worse?

Many factors can lead to acne flares. Sometimes it can be just the change of seasons or moving from one home to another, from one state to another, or from one job to another. Acne can flare from getting married or getting divorced, from losing a loved one, or from having a myriad of other psychologic issues.

Acne can flare from things we put on our skin (from makeup to moisturizers) and from things that we don't use on our skin (from cleansers to creams). Much overlap exists from one person to another in terms of acne triggers, but it is also amazing how different the triggers can be and how many triggers there are.

The following is a list of factors that can cause an acne flare:

- Changing hormone levels in adolescent girls and adult women 2 to 7 days before the menstrual period starts
- Friction caused by leaning on or rubbing the skin
- Pressure from bike helmets, backpacks, or tight collars
- Environmental irritants, such as pollution and high humidity

- Squeezing or picking at blemishes
- Irritation from hard scrubbing of the skin
- Occlusive products that block the opening of the pores
- Poor skin hygiene

19. How can I prevent scarring or help the scars heal faster?

The best way to prevent scars is this: Don't pick at or squeeze your pimples. If you have read any of the other questions, you will have learned that trauma to the skin caused by fingernails or other sharp, non-sterile objects is bad. Your dermatologist is the only person who should extract a blackhead or inject cortisone to help an inflammatory lesion resolve more quickly.

Once an acne lesion is traumatized, it will take longer to heal and will be more likely to leave behind a mark; however, even lesions that are not traumatized can take weeks or months to resolve and can still leave red or brown marks. This is through no direct fault of yours because you didn't pick at it. It usually means, however, that your skin may be more genetically prone to scarring or **hyperpigmentation**. In general, different skin types respond differently to acne during and after a breakout. Breakouts last longer in some people than in others, and some people tend to have red or brown marks left behind for sometimes months after an acne lesion has cleared. This seems to be related to several factors, only some of which are known, such as genetics and skin type. People with fairer skin often seem to complain of red marks that remain red for a long time before they either clear up directly or finally turn brown, whereas those with more olive or darker skin tones note that they start with increased pigmentation

Hyperpigmentation

darkening of skin caused by higher amounts of melanin in a particular spot.

when the acne finally clears. Many people have an overlap with some of both kinds of marks.

The good thing about the red and the brown marks left from acne lesions is that these discolorations are not true scars. Thus, if there is no accompanying scarring, which would be seen as a depression of the skin or change in texture of the skin, the discoloration will usually eventually go away, or lighten significantly over time, or can be treated to expedite the clearing.

Creams that are designed to lighten the skin are available; this can be very useful for hyperpigmentation that results from acne. Laser and other treatments can help the redness. It is also important to try to prevent new lesions and to treat early any lesions that occur to minimize new marks.

The active ingredient in most lightening creams is called **hydroquinone**. Many over-the-counter and prescription formulations containing hydroquinones are available on the market. Some formulations combine hydroquinones with glycolic acid, tretinoin (the active ingredient in Retin-A), sunscreens, **antioxidants**, moisturizers, and many other wonderful ingredients to make their form of hydroquinone better and more appealing. The main difference in over-the-counter versus prescription medications is that the over-the-counter formulations can have a maximum of 2% hydroquinone, whereas the prescription formulations can use up to a 4% concentration of hydroquinone.

Some patients express concern that these lightening agents will bleach all of the color out of the skin. The number one question I get here is, "Will it make me

Acne Overview

Hydroquinone
a class of chemicals that lighten the skin.

Antioxidants
a substance that binds to free radicals, which can damage skin cells, in order to prevent such damage.

look like Michael Jackson?" The answer is not at the concentrations of hydroquinones used in commonly prescribed products on the market. Hydroquinone in high concentrations is cytotoxic to melanocytes. This means that it kills off the pigment-producing cells of the skin. This is why the concentration generally available is a maximum of 4% and patients are advised to use the products only for a specified amount of time, generally 4 to 6 months, before taking a break (Table 6). Other products used to help lighten the skin include licorice extract, yeast ferment, rosmarinic acid, glucosamine, vitamin C, and chamomile extract.

Most of these lightening products contain 2% to 4% hydroquinone along with other agents such as up to 10% glycolic acid, with a sun protection factor (SPF)

Table 6. Prescription Lighteners

Alphaquin HP	Hydroquinone, glycolic acid, sunscreen
Eldopaque Forte	Hydroquinone, sunscreen
Eldoquin Forte	Hydroquinone
Epiquin	Hydroquinone
Glyquin	Hydroquinone, glycolic acid, sunscreen
Lustra	Hydroquinone, glycolic acid
Lustra AF	Hydroquinone, glycolic acid, sunscreen
Melanex	Hydroquinone
Solaquin Forte	Hydroquinone, sunscreen
Tiluma	Hydroquinone, Retin-A, hydrocortisone

of 15 in those containing sunscreen. They come in various forms (from creams to lotion to solutions) in order to make them more appealing to different skin types. Some formulations are more irritating than others. These products take time to work, and results typically begin to be noticeable approximately 1 month after starting treatment.

I generally recommend that the product be used on the entire face or on a larger area as opposed to spot treatment in order to avoid the "halo" effect (a ring of lighter skin around the spot that is usually reversible but can be disconcerting because it can take weeks to months to resolve).

The complications from using hydroquinone products are uncommon and usually have to do with ingredients other than the hydroquinone that are added in to increase absorption of the active ingredient and speed the results. Glycolic acid and retinoids can be irritating to the skin, and sometimes the liquid or gel vehicle itself can be irritating. There is also an uncommon complication from using hydroquinones that is more common in African Americans and with longer-term use of hydroquinones or higher concentrations of the product. This complication, called **exogenous ochronosis,** is a condition of the skin that leaves dark brown or black spots that are mostly in the areas of treatment. It often reverses when the treatment is discontinued but can in some cases be permanent. Another reaction that is more of a concern with the higher concentrations of hydroquinone is permanent and unpredictable bleaching of the skin. This really becomes a concern only when concentrations at 10% or higher of hydroquinone are used for an extended period of time.

Exogenous ochronosis

dark brown or black spots that occur in skin that has been treated with hydroquinones in large doses or for extended periods.

PART TWO

Acne Myths and Facts

Does chocolate cause acne?

Can greasy food or any food cause
or make acne worse?

Does dirty skin make acne worse?

More ...

20. Does chocolate cause acne?

Many myths exist about what causes acne. Chocolate and greasy foods are often blamed, but exactly what effect foods seem to have on either the development or the course of acne in most people remains unclear. No studies have been able to show that chocolate affects acne.

In a study looking at the possible effects of chocolate, particularly on acne, it was shown that chocolate had no effect on most patients. In a few, it made the acne worse, and in a few others, it made their acne better. I have many patients who insist, however, that they are sure that their acne flares when they eat chocolate. These patients may have an overlap of acne and another condition that can sometimes look like acne, called rosacea.

Most commonly, I get parents who come in with their teenager insisting that chocolate causes acne and looking to me for reinforcement of this myth. Meanwhile, I see the child rolling his or her eyes and probably wishing that he or she were anywhere but in my office. I do my best to tell the facts as we know them today, but in the end, I know that it is difficult to break this cycle of misinformation. All I can offer is this: "If you think the chocolate makes you break out, don't eat the chocolate."

21. Can greasy food or any food cause or make acne worse?

As with chocolate, studies have not been able to show any association between acne flares and greasy foods. It does seem that all of the foods implicated in causing acne are tasty. This includes such delicacies as chocolate, candy, nuts, soda, fried foods, and orange juice. I think that over the years everything has been suggested to cause acne—from water to nearly any food you can imagine.

The reality is that there is no scientific evidence available to show that high-carbohydrate and/or fat intake has any effect on sebum production or acne. Part of the problem is that there are so many factors that can cause acne to get worse that it is very difficult to isolate a single factor and prove that it does or does not affect this condition.

For many years, dairy foods have been linked to acne, and there have been reports that acne patients who have limited or eliminated milk consumption have experienced substantial improvement in their acne. Results from two studies done at Harvard Medical School seem to validate those reports. They provided 6,500 teenage boys and girls, ranging in age from 8–14 years old, who are part of an ongoing larger, broader study, with questionnaires regarding their acne and milk/dairy consumption. Both studies showed a significant positive association between milk consumption and acne according to the authors of the study. The results were independent of the fat content of the milk, with "whole," "reduced fat," and "skim" milk all showing statistically significant associations with acne. There were also increased association with acne and milk-based instant breakfast drinks, sherbet, cottage cheese, and cream cheese, but not with other dairy foods or with other foods such as French fries, chocolate, candy, or pizza. In the study, girls were more affected than boys. It may be that the hormones which are produced naturally in the milk of cows, particularly pregnant cows, which makes up between 75% and 90% of marketed milk and dairy products, plays an important role. Milk provides an important source of calcium and protein for many in this age group and special care needs to be taken to ensure that there is adequate calcium in the diet if a dairy-free diet is attempted.

It may be that certain situations or stressors that make those foods more tempting or harder to resist at any given time may be the ultimate culprit for acne flares. In the meantime, if you feel that a certain food makes the acne worse for you in particular, you should try to avoid that food, within reason. You clearly won't benefit from being malnourished, but I have never heard of anyone becoming malnourished from giving up high-fat, high-carbohydrate junk food or most of the foods that people most commonly complain of as being a cause of acne flares.

One ingredient that can make acne worse, if eaten in large enough quantities, is iodine. Foods that are high in iodine, such as seaweed and other seafood, if eaten in a large enough volume can have an effect on acne.

22. Does dirty skin make acne worse?

Another common myth is that dirty skin causes acne. Dirt does not cause blackheads and other acne lesions; however, poor skin hygiene can make acne worse. Proper skin hygiene is very important in maintaining healthy skin. It not only helps control acne by working from the outside to help reduce buildup of skin cells around the pores, it also helps to keep the skin healthy and looking its best even at the deeper layers.

Proper skin hygiene is very important in maintaining healthy skin.

On the other hand, over-washing can be very unhealthy for the skin and is usually a bigger problem than not washing enough. Using drying, harsh soaps on the skin on a regular basis can strip away the skin's natural, healthy barrier and leave it more vulnerable to infection and irritation. It can leave the skin red and actually cause a rash that mimics acne.

The squeaky-clean feel that used to be considered a good thing is really a sign that you have overdone it and need to moisturize. Choose a soap-free cleanser for the face, as soaps contain a class of ingredients called **surfactants**, which give the soap its marvelous lather. Surfactant's job is to bind to oils and remove them from your skin, leaving your skin clean in the process. The problem is that they are irritating to the skin and remove more oils than you need to have removed.

Surfactants
chemicals that lower the surface tension of a liquid, allowing easier spreading; they are often used in soaps and detergents.

Instead, you can try a gentle exfoliating cleanser at night to remove the dirt and makeup. In the morning, it is generally better for most people to use a gentle soap-free cleanser, one that may not even create any lather, followed by your usual morning routine of sunscreen and any other regimen that you may follow.

23. Does stress affect acne?

Although stress does not directly cause acne, it is one of the factors that makes acne worse. Different people handle stress differently—some lose their hair, others get ulcers, whereas still others get migraines or have other physical or psychologic side effects. Basically, stress can make any condition worse. There are excellent ways to manage stressful situations, which can have profound effects in the treatment of acne.

Maria's comments:

I am a 20-year-old woman in college. I also work part time to try to earn some extra money to pay for school, and I help my sister take care of her young child. Every time I have an exam at school, my acne flares big time. My face looks like a pizza pie, and I have to try really hard not to pick at the pimples. I know that if I pick, the marks will get redder and be more likely to scar, but sometimes I can't help myself. I just want the skin to feel smooth. One thing that I have found to help me is to increase the acne treatments before exams begin and to treat the acne more often. I have one regimen for in-between exams and another regimen that is stronger for when I have exams. This helps make it so I have fewer pimples, and they go away faster. It also gives me something to do besides pick at the zits.

When people are under stress they do things differently: They eat different foods, usually foods that are higher in fat and sugar. They sleep less, and the quality of the sleep that they do get is generally poor. They also react to situations differently, getting angry more easily and maybe picking at their skin more, or being less compliant with their acne treatment regimens. Hormones called cortisols are released in times of stress. These hormones were very helpful in primitive times in helping us survive life-threatening situations. They are known as the "fight or flight" reactions. The release of these hormones puts the body on high alert. Our palms sweat, the heart rate increases, and all of our energy becomes available in one blast to get us through the immediate, threatening stressor.

This was fine, even necessary, in the days when so much that happened was a matter of life or death. Now, when it comes to stressors that we currently experience, chances are that we do not need such high levels of cortisols to see us through. But that is what we get. In response to the stressor, whether it is an exam or meeting or date or any other perceived good or bad factor, we release the same hormones, cortisols. The longer-term effects of increased cortisols are suppression of the immune system and, of course, acne, as the *P. acnes* bacteria flourishes in the depressed immune state.

Stress management is an important part of treatment for acne. It helps to anticipate situations that are stressful to you and to try to work through them as best as you can in order to minimize the effect of the stress on your body and mind. This not only helps to keep your skin clear but also helps in every part of your life. I am a big fan of relaxation techniques. I find that they are very helpful in clearing the mind and controlling stress.

Stress management is an important part of acne treatment.

A simple technique is one in which you slowly take in a deep breath, hold it for 4 seconds, and then slowly breathe out. As you slowly exhale, feel your entire body relax and the positive energy return to your body. Obviously, you should not do this while driving or in other situations that require your full attention, but it can be very useful to take a few seconds before a big meeting or in the middle of an exam or even on a long night of studying. It is amazing to me how little we focus on the importance of breathing and the power of our minds to help guide us in the right directions.

It is also helpful to be more aggressive in your acne treatment in these circumstances. This will help minimize the severity of the acne and clear the skin more quickly.

Maria's comments:

Every time I have a school exam or if I feel pulled in too many directions at once, I get sick. It starts with my diet. I

can't find the time to get a real meal, so I just grab some-
thing here and there, usually from the school vending
machine. I end up staying up late, drinking tons of coffee to
cram for the exam, and then I am exhausted for days. I
start getting headaches and then stuffiness and sometimes
even a fever. When the acne comes a few days later, it just
makes the whole situation worse. I have found that, along
with adjusting my acne treatment routine, I try to plan
ahead for exams. I cook a few meals in advance and freeze
them so that I can microwave a meal quickly when I need
it. Also, I try to drink more water along with my coffee.
This has made a big difference for me. The exams are still
hard. I still feel a lot of pressure to do too much in too little
time; however, I don't make myself sick over it, and my
acne is much, much better.

Some people get stressed more easily than others. It is
very important to try to manage the stressors in your
life and to minimize them as much as possible in order
to help maintain control of acne, as well as for your
overall well-being.

24. Why does my acne get better/worse when I go in the sun or tanning salon?

For some people, especially those with inflammatory
acne, there is a dramatic improvement in the skin over
the summer, when the days are longer and we typically
spend more time outdoors, or after sun exposure. This
may be because of ingredients called porphyrins that
are part of the *P. acnes* bacteria. These porphyrins are
very sensitive to sunlight, especially in the 410–420
nm range (see Question 89). This would be in the area
of violet/blue light (see Table 7). Ultraviolet light
(UVA and UVB) is invisible. However, it is damaging

Table 7. Spectrum of Light

Type of light	Wavelength
UVB	290–320
UVA	320–400
Visible	400–700
Violet	400–430
Blue	430–500
Green	500–560
Yellow to orange	560–620
Orange to red	620–700

to the skin in many ways. It is well known to cause premature aging of the skin and various types of skin cancer. It is also known to make acne worse. It is also known to be comedogenic.

Sun exposure has a drying effect on the skin and damages the sebaceous glands, making them temporarily less active. For this reason, people with overactive sebaceous glands may find that their skin gets initially better after sun exposure; however, the heat and sweating that often accompany sun exposure can make acne worse for some people. Sun exposure also greatly increases the risks of skin cancer and premature aging of the skin.

Some people go to tanning salons thinking that this is a safe way to get "sun" and to treat their acne. Tanning beds contain the same **ultraviolet radiation** found in natural sunlight; however, there is a higher amount of

Ultraviolet radiation
light emitted by the sun that can have damaging effects on skin.

Table 8.   UV in Natural and Artificial Light

	Natural Light	Tanning Beds
Ultraviolet A	90%	95%
Ultraviolet B	10%	5%

ultraviolet A than in natural sunlight and less ultraviolet B than found in nature (Table 8).

Prolonged exposure to ultraviolet light may actually increase comedonal acne. In addition, many studies show that tanning beds are not safe. Chronic sun exposure from any source, including tanning beds, increases the risk of skin cancer and premature aging. Also, it is well known scientifically that sun exposure is immunosuppressive to the skin and slows wound healing. Specifically, **collagen** formation is affected, which means that the marks left behind from any healing lesions will take longer to disappear and will even have a higher chance of leaving a permanent scar.

Collagen

the main protein in the deeper layers of skin. It is responsible for the elasticity of the skin and plays a prominent role in development of scars.

Avoid excessive sun exposure in general and tanning beds in particular, especially if you have acne.

The bottom line here is very clearly to avoid excessive sun exposure in general and tanning beds in particular, especially if you have acne. This is the best way to keep your skin looking younger, more healthy, and radiant. If you like the look of a suntan, try the sunless tanning products that are now available. They are safe and create a very natural-looking "tan" without the damage of sun exposure.

Hundreds of products are available that offer a quick, easy way to get the color of a suntan you want without the sun damage. The active ingredient in sunless tanners is dihydroxyacetone, or DHA. This is a simple nontoxic ingredient that stains the upper layers of the skin to create brown or golden brown compounds. Most self-tanners have concentrations of between 2% and 5% DHA. The deeper the tanning product, the more concentrated the DHA. Other ingredients may be added in as well, such as sunscreen and fragrance to make products more enticing.

The more you use the sunless tanners, the better you get at applying them evenly, which means that there will be less of a problem with streak marks or other problems from unevenness of the application. There are also salons and spas that offer "bronzing" sessions at a relatively reasonable price (usually less expensive than the cost of a tanning session).

Many of the tanning salons are getting smart and are starting to offer these treatments for clients who want the color without the damage. Just be careful not to get talked into a tanning bed treatment instead. The sunless tanning machines at these sites offer shower-type "spray-on" booths that you stand in for less than 1 minute and walk out with an even coating of the product. Sessions have to be repeated about once a week.

25. Can my sunscreen make me break out?

Another myth is that sunscreens cause acne. For people who feel that they breakout after using sunscreens, it may be that they are having an irritant reaction to the sunscreen or to the sun that can look like acne. These types of rashes can have the red bumps that look just like acne but don't typically improve with acne medications.

The best treatment is to avoid the irritant, whether it is the sun or the products with which you have reacted.

If the rash persists, allergy testing can be done; this sometimes helps to identify the offending agent. This is done by using patch testing of common offending agents to the skin. Sometimes specific tests can be done if a particular agent is thought to be the culprit.

Finally, it may be that the vehicle of the sunscreen preparation, not the active ingredient of the sunscreen itself, may be too greasy or occlusive, and therefore a different choice of sunscreen should be made. If you are using a cream, switch to a lotion. If you are using a lotion, try a gel. Sunscreens are also available in oil-free preparations for those with especially oily or acne-prone skin.

For my younger patients with oilier skin, I usually recommend a sunscreen in a gel formulation. I find that the gel dries more quickly and does not run into the eyes in those who are more physically active and may be sweating more. I also find that gels, because they are more drying, are less likely to be a problem for those with acne.

There are wonderful SPF-tinted moisturizers that help to conceal the acne while protecting from the sun. Products are available that combine acne treatments with sun protection, which can also be useful. Many new combination sunscreen/treatments are available in nearly every type of vehicle, and thus there most likely is something for everyone.

26. How can I have acne at my age (past my teenage years)?

This is the most commonly asked question that I get in my office regarding acne. Undoubtedly, every patient I see who is over 18 who comes in with acne, either recurrent or for the first time, seems to be personally insulted that they are afflicted with this dreaded condition. They want to know how they can have acne at their age and why their acne was never this bad when they were teenagers. How could they have acne now when they never even had any acne at all as a teenager?

Lisa's comments:

I don't know what happened to me. I made it through my teenage years with perfect skin, and now I wake up at 35 feeling like a kid just going through puberty. My skin is sometimes oily and sometimes dry, but either way it is always breaking out. At first I thought I must be mistaken. I never even thought it was possible to have acne at my age. I tried washing more often and changing my makeup, but that didn't help. Next I tried picking the pimples, but they looked horrible and left scars. Worst of all, I kept getting new pimples anyway! All of the treatments I found at the drug store seemed to be very drying, and they all seemed to be aimed at teenagers. I felt silly and embarrassed just being there. I need to look good for my job, and I try to have an active social life. It has been very depressing to be breaking out at my age.

One of the greatest myths about acne is that is occurs in only teenagers and that if you can get through those years you are home free. The reality is that acne in adults is a very common occurrence and needs to be addressed.

One of the greatest myths about acne is that is occurs in only teenagers.

For some, acne does not begin or become a significant issue until sometime after their teenage years. In teens and preteens, acne starts as mostly comedones in the central area of the face—the forehead, nose, and cheeks. Over the next few months to years, as the hormonal influences kick in, the acne takes on more variations and can be inflammatory as well. These hormonal influences sometimes don't take effect until later in teenage years or even later into our 20s or 30s and occasionally even later in life.

For those in whom the hormones have an early effect during adolescence, there is no guarantee that the hormones responsible will slow down or have less of an influence over time. Accompanied by all of the other factors that affect us over time, such as exams, work, family and friends, there can be lots of excuses for acne to persist for many, many—always too many—years.

Lisa's comments:

I noticed that my acne occurred mostly on my chin and on the sides of my neck. A lot of the pimples stayed under the skin and never seemed to come up to the surface, so I couldn't even get at them if I wanted to. There was also a lot of redness on my chin, especially in the areas around the pimples. When I wore makeup, it just seemed to make my skin look bumpy, although it did help cover the redness.

The acne that occurs in adults often has a different distribution than it does in teenage acne. Adult acne tends to center more on the lower part of the face, around the chin, and along the jaw line. It is much more common in women than in men and can be more difficult to control because the skin in this area is often more sensitive and more easily irritated from the often drying medications that are used in acne.

Lisa's comments:

I was so relieved when my acne finally started to improve. I took an antibiotic by mouth for about 3 months, and now

I take it every now and then for a month if I have a difficult flare. I started an oral contraceptive since I am not planning pregnancy any time soon, and I also use a sulfa-based face wash and use a retinoid on a regular basis. I feel like I got my skin back. What a relief!

It is also important for women to consider whether they are currently pregnant or planning pregnancy in the near future when considering different treatment options because some medications should not be used in these situations. There can be a lot of trial and error in trying to get control of the acne in this population, with oral antibiotics and combinations of topical medications being especially useful. Many of these women often find that starting an oral contraceptive pill is the best therapy, sometimes getting them to the point where they don't need topical treatments at all, or only occasionally at worst.

27. Do medications cause acne?

There is a long list of medications that list acne as a possible side effect. The list includes classes of drugs including androgens, **lithium**, potassium iodide, some oral contraceptives, and other medications. This does not mean that you should never take these medications if your physician prescribes them. It does mean that you should discuss your concerns regarding this side effect and consider alternate treatments (if available) should the acne become problematic. The acne from medications is generally similar to acne from other causes and is treated with the same medications. The difference is that it may take longer to gain control of the acne (Table 9).

Lithium

a chemical element often used as a mood stabilizer.

Table 9.   Medications That May Aggravate Acne

Corticosteroids
Estrogens
Halodol/antipsychotic medications
Isoniazid
Lithium
Dilantin
Potassium iodide
Quinine
Testosterone

28. Does makeup cause acne?

Greasy, thick cosmetics may alter the cells of the follicles and make them stick together more easily, producing a plug that is the beginning step in the onset of a pimple. A big and continuing trend toward oil-free everything exists as a way to prevent acne; however, different kinds of "oils" can be found in products that may or may not make acne worse.

Certain "oils/fats/lipids" are naturally found in the skin that keep it healthy and help maintain important functions, mainly as a barrier against insults from the outside world. Such protection would include helping the skin function as an effective barrier, which means it would effectively block bacteria from penetrating the skin, prevent water loss from the skin, and improve water retention within the skin to keep it looking healthy and supple. Many companies have made products that contain these "essential lipids" to not only keep the skin healthy but also to keep it looking its best.

The oils that are problematic are some of those that are produced by the sebaceous glands or certain heavier types, such as mineral oil. These oils leave the skin looking shiny and can be aggravating to acne. Many products are specifically tested, now mostly in only laboratory settings and on humans, for their ability to cause or worsen acne. Once they pass this test, they are labeled "non-comedogenic" or "non-acnegenic."

Many of the acne-control products available are in many ways sebaceous oil-control products. Unfortunately, a negative result of testing different batches of ingredients is that results have not been consistent, which means that the batch you are using may be more, or less, comedogenic. Also, the exact comedogenic potential of any product is not known. It is impossible to take into account all of the interactions with all the individual comedogenic and noncomedogenic ingredients included in the final mixture of the product. You have to look at your own skin and see how you tolerate certain products. Simply knowing the ingredients is not enough to make an accurate predication about whether a product will be **acnegenic**. Physical characteristics of the product, such as the density and oiliness, are also not predictive of an acnegenic response. Finally, to add to the confusion, cosmetics that do not contain comedogenic agents are not guaranteed to be noncomedogenic.

In recommending cosmetics to my acne-prone patients I try to give them guidelines from which they can make their own decisions as to which products would be best for them. Start with keeping it simple: Choose products that have 10 or fewer ingredients. In choosing foundations, look for loose powders since they help

Acnegenic

products that induce inflammatory lesions (e.g. papules, pustules) to form, usually within 2 to 3 days of using the product.

absorb excess oil from the skin. If you use a liquid foundation, look for ones that are silicone (dimethicone, cyclomethicone) based since this ingredient sits very smoothly on the skin and is nongreasy, nonacnegenic, and noncomedogenic. Try to avoid cosmetics that contain D&C red dyes since these dyes are highly comedogenic. It can be difficult to find the right blush without D&C red dyes.

Finally, don't assume that just because a product is "natural" it is better for your skin. The word *natural* is undefined and unregulated, and even products that are labeled "all-natural" may include ingredients that are comedogenic and acnegenic.

Many acne treatments are drying or otherwise irritating to the skin, and in these cases, a more emollient or creamier moisturizer may be indicated, especially in the evening before bed because water loss from the skin is increased at night while you are sleeping.

29. Does exercise affect acne?

Some people notice that their acne gets worse after exercise, especially on the back. It helps to apply acne treatment medications before your workout and to shower immediately after the workout. The inflammatory type of acne is most common here. This means that topical antibiotics are helpful, especially when used along with a topical BP. Just be careful with the leave-on topical BPs because they are known to cause bleaching of fabrics and can ruin your workout clothing. As a good alternative, you can try using BP and/or salicylic acid cleansers after the workout.

It is unclear the exact effect exercise has on bringing out acne. It may be a combination of factors such as increased sweat combined with sticky surface skin cells leading to blockage of the pores, or it may be the heat combined with friction that activates the *P. acnes* bacteria in some people. It may be that exercise, heat, and sweat lead to increased activity of the sebaceous glands, which are the oil-producing glands in the skin. They are attached to the hair follicles and are especially prominent on the face and upper back. The sebum produced by the sebaceous glands is food for the *P. acnes* bacteria that also live at the base of the follicles. The increased food supply may lead to more active *P. acnes* with the final result of more acne.

30. Should I use only oil-free products on my skin if I am prone to acne?

The definition of "oil free" is more complicated that it first seems. All oil-free products avoid most ingredients that contain the actual word "oil" in their name, such as "mineral oil." However, plenty of ingredients do not have the literal word "oil" in their name, such as glyceryl tribehenate or lanolin. Also, there are some ingredients—waxes such as carnauba and oily hydrocarbons such as petrolatum and squalene—that are not oils but should not be included in an oil-free product. The skin-care industry is not always clear or strict in avoiding these ingredients in oil-free formulations. Essential oils, such as those used as fragrance, are not a problem in that they do not behave as other oils and can be used in the oil-free formulations.

Oil-free products can be divided into two groups. The first contains strictly oil-free products, which are usually drying. There are some excellent exceptions in that ingredients such as propylene glycol, glycerin, and silicone bases are not oils and are not drying. For people with acne that is resistant to treatment, it is very helpful to identify products that are strictly oil free to complement their topical therapy. These products include solutions, gels, and emulsions of oil-free ingredients. Ingredients such as fatty acids, fatty alcohols, sterols, and silicones are acceptable in strictly oil-free preparations. The second group consists of borderline oil-free products that contain oil-like emollients called **esters**. Some are not technically considered to be oils or fats but are oil-like in the way that they affect the skin. For example, many of the ingredients that have been classified as comedogenic are emollient esters. Oil-free emulsions of emollient esters and water are weakly moisturizing and are best used by people with slightly oily to slightly dry skin that want additional moisturizing.

Esters

oil-like emollients sometimes found in skin-care products.

Powders absorb water and oil, which shifts the skin toward more dry from more oily. Many powders are modified to make them less drying and more cosmetically acceptable for people with a wider range of skin issues.

31. Why do movie and rock stars or other famous people never seem to have acne?

Two reasons for this exist: (1) They see their dermatologists often, and (2) they wear a lot of makeup. When your income depends on how you look, you tend to take better care of your skin. Models and actors are often meticulous about their skin care. They understand more than most how important it is to keep their skin looking good, and they are much more likely to have a rigorous skin care routine to keep their skin looking polished and smooth.

PART THREE

When to Treat

I get only a few pimples each month.
Do I need to treat them?

Why do I always get acne in the same spots?

Do I need a blood test to evaluate my acne?

More . . .

32. I get only a few pimples each month. Do I need to treat them?

Whether to treat acne at all and even how to treat acne are very personal decisions. Some people are devastated by one lesion, especially if it is centered right in the middle of their nose; others can have many lesions and barely even notice. I have learned in my practice never to guess why someone has come in for the visit. I arrived at this conclusion after several instances of sitting down, looking at the patient, and saying, "So, you are here for your acne?" thinking that without a doubt, the acne was the reason for the visit—only to be shot down with, "No, I'm here for this mole on my arm." Clearly, some are more bothered by their acne than others.

Acne is divided into three basic categories from mild to severe depending on the number of pimples and the amount of scarring:

1. mild = nonscarring, fewer than 10 lesions;

2. moderate = may scar, more than 10 lesions; and

3. severe = cystic, nodulocystic, scarring.

If you get only one new acne lesion of any type per month but each lesion leaves behind a scar, this would make 12 new scars each year. In this case, it would be wise to treat the acne in order to prevent as many new lesions as possible and to help the ones that do appear to clear as quickly as possible in order to minimize the chance of permanent scarring.

It is also important to remember to avoid picking at or squeezing lesions. I will say this 100 times throughout this book, if I haven't already. Don't pick. **DO NOT**

PICK. Picking is bad. Picking at acne lesions or scars leads to a longer duration of lesions and a higher chance of permanent scarring as well as increased pain at the site (see Questions 12 and 13).

Amanda's comments:

I have been thinking about acne for it seems like forever. I tried everything over the counter before going to the doctor. I tried herbal supplements and changes in my diet. At first I thought that my diet really made a big difference. I gave up sugar. I became a vegetarian, and I drank a ton of water. I followed some diet I found on the Internet, and then I tried two or three more. After a while, no matter what I did, I kept getting new pimples. I couldn't believe that at age 28 I could still be breaking out like a teenager. Actually, my acne got to a point where it was even worse than when I was a teenager. I found I was avoiding social situations, and I was not as outgoing at work either. Because I am in sales, my appearance is very important to my job. Also, I take really good care of myself, so I want my skin look its best. I spend a lot of time looking at my skin, and I don't like what I see. I also spend a lot of time looking up products, both on the Internet and in the stores. There is so much to choose from that sometimes it gets overwhelming. It helped a lot to use prescription acne medications from my doctor and to review with her the products I am using from the store. We also reviewed both products and ingredients that are better for my skin type and that would work well with the prescription medications I am using. I still get a few pimples here and there, but not nearly as many, and they go away more quickly—never quickly enough, though. I have a much better sense of my skin and what works for me. That gives me a lot more confidence, which has made a big difference in both my job and my life in general.

There are four factors to consider in deciding when to treat and how to treat acne. They are as follows:

- What is the severity of the lesions present? How long do the pimples last, and are they very itchy or painful?
- How long has the acne been a problem? Is it a recent occurrence that you can relate to specific events—such as a specific medication you took for a while, or a new product you are using—or has it been going on for years?
- How have you responded to treatment in the past?
- What is the tendency for scarring and hyperpigmentation? Do they leave behind red or brown marks or scars?

You can make a list for yourself as to these four factors. This will help guide you as to whether you might need treatment, and it will help your doctor decide the right treatment plan for you.

33. Why do I always get acne in the same spots?

For so many people, it seems that acne lesions recur in the same spot or spots every time the pimples come back. This is sometimes on a monthly basis for women, which often coincides with their periods. For others, it seems to occur at random.

Dawn's comments:

I am a nurse, and I am constantly on the phone when I am at work. I share the phone with others at the nurse's station, and no matter how much I try to keep the phone clean by wiping it with alcohol swabs I know that it is not enough.

I don't think it is a coincidence that I get acne on the right side of my face where the receiver touches my skin. The area is now starting to have scarring and discoloration.

When acne recurs regularly in the same spot, there may be several explanations. It may be that there is a weakness of the follicular wall in the spot that keeps breaking out. There may also be local hormonal fluctuations in the skin. Some people touch their skin in the same spot, and that constant touching can also be a factor. Rarely is dirt from contact from a phone or other substance the cause of recurrent acne.

It may be that if the object is left on the skin for long periods of time, occlusion or moisture and irritation may develop; however, acne is not contagious because the bacteria that causes the inflammatory form of acne is deep at the base of the follicle and is not accessible to the upper layers of the skin from which it might be transferred. There are, however, other types of bacterial infections, such as staphylococcal or streptococcal infections, that could, at least hypothetically, be transferred and that could cause a rash that mimics acne.

34. Do I need a blood test to evaluate my acne?

Acne is a condition of the skin. In general, blood tests are not usually indicated for people with acne unless certain conditions related to hormonal imbalance are suspected. In these cases, there may be excessive androgen production from either the adrenal gland or the ovary. In these cases, the workup often includes the measurement of selective androgens in the blood that are produced by these glands.

It is important to note that most people with acne do not typically have significant hormonal abnormalities. This does not mean that hormones are not affecting the acne; it simply means that the body is not overproducing hormones. There may be oversensitivity at the level of the sebaceous gland to the normal amounts of circulating hormones. It is has been shown that both hormonal and nonhormonal therapies that reduce sebum production may be very useful in treating acne.

The clue that hormonal treatments might be an appropriate option for a woman, even in the face of normal blood tests, is acne that is unresponsive or only minimally responsive to conventional oral and topical acne treatments, or if the acne recurs very quickly after stopping oral antibiotics. Hormonal treatments are generally used only in women because of the unacceptable feminizing effects that they would have on men.

35. When should I ask my internist or primary care physician to send me to a specialist?

If you feel that your acne is persistent or is leading to scarring and you have tried what you consider to be a reasonable treatment course with over-the-counter and/or prescription medications, you may want to consider consulting a dermatologist for your acne. Dermatologists are medical doctors who specialize in all conditions of the skin, hair, and nails. Some insurance plans require referrals from the primary care physician. In these cases, you may need to request a referral in order to have your insurance cover the visits.

Dermatologists specialize in the treatment of acne, as well as many other skin conditions, and are most likely to be aware of the latest trends in treatment options to help control the acne as quickly as possible; however, not everyone needs to see a doctor to have his or her acne treated. Many people with mild acne do very well with over-the-counter treatments that are widely available. In fact, most people have tried at least one or several over-the-counter or prescription treatments before consulting a dermatologist.

36. How often should I wash my face?

It is important to keep the face clean without over-washing or scrubbing. The face, or any skin that is overwashed, will be more easily irritated and may look red or even have cuts in it. Sometimes the result can be an irritant **dermatitis** that mimics acne. If the skin is then treated with medications designed to treat acne, the rash can actually worsen and start a negative cycle that remains unresponsive or is worsened by acne treatments. The solution in these cases is to wash less often—no more than once or twice a day—and to use gentle, surfactant-free gentle cleansers followed by a facial moisturizer.

The approach to washing should depend on your level of physical activity, whether your skin tends to be oily or dry, and the amount of time that you are willing to put into thinking about it. In general, washing in the evening is more important than washing in the morning. Products you use may vary depending on the season. More gentle, moisturizing products may be more appropriate in the winter months, with only occasional exfoliation, while more drying, foaming cleansers and more frequent exfoliation may be better for the warmer, more humid summer season.

When to Treat

Keep the face clean without overwashing.

Dermatitis
inflammation or irritation of the skin.

Cleansers may also serve different purposes. Some are designed simply to rid the skin of accumulated sebum and to remove makeup and daily dirt, whereas others are more aggressive with the goal of exfoliation of the dead upper layers of the skin. Still others are medicated to specifically treat acne while cleansing.

A variety of cleansers are available, from foaming washes that are more drying, and potentially more irritating, to nonlathering cleansing milks that are the least irritating but usually provide little in the way of lather. Some cleansers have microbeads of various sizes and consistencies to exfoliate while they clean, and finally, some come already packaged in cleansing cloths that may or may not require the addition of water before use, which makes them especially convenient for those who travel. The medicated cleansers generally contain BP or salicylic acid or **α-hydroxy acid** in a variety of concentrations or sulfa-type ingredients.

α-hydroxy acids

naturally occurring acids, derived from the sugars in particular plants, that are sometimes used in skin care products to promote turnover of dead skin cells.

In general, washing in the evening is more important that washing in the morning. Also, exfoliating cleansers are useful for all but the most sensitive skin types, but I usually recommend that they be used only once or twice a week or less depending on the other products being used and the sensitivity of the skin. For some people, the only acne treatment that they need may be found in the cleanser.

For people who are easily irritated by topical BP-based products, a BP cleanser may be the ideal option for acne treatment. It is left on for only a few minutes before being rinsed, followed by a face moisturizer, therefore making the likelihood for irritation low; however, the BP is still effective in its ability to reduce the amount of bacteria in the skin, even when left on the skin for such short periods of time, and thereby helps treat the acne with minimal irritation.

Patients with acne tend to wash their skin excessively in an attempt to reduce oiliness. No scientific evidence states that the lack of washing is associated with acne or that frequent washing improves the condition. It is known that too vigorous cleansing and scrubbing can aggravate the inflammatory phase of acne. Normal washing does not affect the reservoir of lipids (fats/oils) in the follicle, which is the site where the problem originates. Furthermore, antibacterial soaps that contain agents such as **triclosan** and **chlorhexidine** do not affect *P. acnes*. In addition, these soaps can be irritating.

For these reasons, antibacterial soaps are not indicated in acne. The exception is the benzoyl peroxide wash, which does suppress and even kills *P. acnes*, even when used as a cleanser; however, overcleansing, even with BP, can be irritating to the skin and should be avoided.

37. Are facials good for my skin?

Aestheticians in salons and spas usually perform facials. They are less commonly provided by aestheticians in a doctor's office. There are a variety in terms of different types of procedures offered and expertise on the part of the facialist. A typical facial takes about 30 to 45 minutes and consists of a series of steps starting with cleansing the skin, massage, heat wraps, extraction of blackheads, and application of creams.

There are now a variety of different types of facials, from oxygen facials to vitamin C facials to "gold" facials and much more. These can be very relaxing and soothing to the skin, and some people find them to be therapeutic.

When to Treat

Triclosan
a potent wide-spectrum antibacterial and antifungal agent.

Chlorhexidine
a broad-spectrum anti-microbial agent sometimes used in antibacterial soaps.

Aesthetician
a person trained to improve the appearance of skin through facial massage, application of skincare products or cosmetics, heat wraps, and similar techniques that affect only the skin surface.

A few areas exist, however, where I am concerned about potential problems with facials. One concern is any sensitivity that you may have to any of the creams or lotions used, which can lead to an irritant reaction. Another concern is with the expertise of the person performing the facial—an overly aggressive facial, especially if done by an improperly trained or inexperienced technician, can leave your face worse than when you began. My main concern, however, is with the extraction part of the facial. In this part of the procedure, the facialist often uses a tissue paper and his or her fingernails or other instrument to squeeze the pores or whiteheads or blackheads to extract the contents. This can lead to redness and swelling and is only a temporary improvement because the pore will only fill again over the next few days. I have seen scarring and redness that can last for months after this type of extraction.

If you are considering having a facial, get referrals from your dermatologist or friends who have had facials and ask questions before you trust your face to anyone. Also, consider just skipping the extraction part of the facial, at least until you get comfortable with the technician. The other part of the service that you really have to beware of is that the technicians will try to sell you a lot of products before you leave.

Consider making a list of the products that they recommend and asking your dermatologist about them. Try only one new product at a time, adding a new product approximately every 2 weeks so that in case you have an irritation from any given product, it will be easier to identify and eliminate that product before trying anything else.

PART FOUR

Topical Acne Treatment

What different types of topical treatments
are available for acne?

How long should it take to see results?

Why are there so many different treatments for acne?

More ...

38. What different types of topical treatments are available for acne?

Many wonderful topical treatments are available for acne, both over the counter and prescription. As for the over-the-counter treatments, the formulations are designed to work on many different levels. First, there is the packaging, because so much of selling a product comes from getting you to believe that it is the best product available. Once the company has your attention, they want you to keep buying the product, and thus, they often make a variety of formulations based on the same theme. They may offer a BP wipe, gel, cream, foam, and BP wash of various strengths. They may offer salicylic acid in a wash, lotion, makeup, or other formulation to allow them to claim 8- to 12-hour shine control. The idea is to offer the product in as many formulations as possible to appeal to as wide an audience as possible. There is often special attention to the way the product feels and looks on the skin and to covering the acne while treating it. These products have become increasingly more sophisticated over the years and have contributed very nicely to the arena of acne treatment.

The larger companies especially do a lot of research on what the acne treatment-seeking population is looking for, and they will find a way to get it to you as best as they can. There are limits to what the over-the-counter market can offer and claim; treatments alone are often not enough to address the issues of acne completely, especially in cases of moderate or severe acne. They are often excellent when used along with prescription medications.

The focus of prescription topical treatments is to decrease the amount of bacteria present in the skin, improve skin cell turnover to minimize microcomedo formation, and improve the redness and inflammation associated with acne. Prescription medications are often combinations of one or more active ingredients, and the claims that they can make generally go further than claims from over-the-counter treatments. Medications are also available that are used to reduce the brown spots (known as hyperpigmentation) that can be left behind after the acne lesions have cleared (Table 10). But, even after the acne is cleared your job is not over. Most people need a maintenance program to help prevent new acne lesions from forming and keep their skin clear over the long term.

39. How long should it take to see results?

I see plenty of patients who come in with a list of treatments that they have tried and that have reportedly failed. When I question them further, I commonly learn that they gave the medicine only 1 or 2 weeks before giving up and deciding that the treatment was not working. It is very important to realize that although results can sometimes begin in as little as 1 week, it often takes 4 to 6 weeks to really see significant improvement. It is important to continue the regimen for at least the full 6 weeks before you decide that the treatment is not working for you.

Initially, you should notice the pimples drying up. They can leave red marks behind that can last for days to weeks to months. The red marks are not affected by the acne treatments because they are simply remnants of the acne that was present earlier, rather than active acne, and they should not be confused with true acne lesions. They should be touched or picked at as little as possible to allow the skin to recover more quickly.

Table 10. Topical Treatments

Benzoyl peroxide

2% to 10%—cream, gel, cleanser, and pads
Combination with antibiotics
BP 4.5% or 8.5% in emollient 10% urea base—cream, gel, and cleanser

Antibiotics

Erythromycin
Clindamycin

Retinoids

Retin-A
Differin
Tazorac

Azelaic acid

Azelex
Finacea

Hydroxy acids

α-Hydroxy acid (glycolic acid)
β-Hydroxy acid (salicylic acid)

Hydroquinones

Combined with Retin A and hydrocortisone

Combination treatments

BP/erythromycin
BP/clindamycin
BP/urea (emollient)
RA/hydroquinone/hydrocortisone

With continued treatment, the next thing that you should notice is that you get fewer new lesions and that the lesions that do appear clear more quickly with less redness or scarring, if any. Over the next few months, the red marks may turn brown before they disappear, or fading creams can be prescribed to help them fade faster.

Compliance is key to getting results. If you don't use the medication as directed, for whatever reason, it will take longer to get results. Also, if you use too much medication or apply it too often, you increase the risk of irritation, which will also make your skin look less than optimal. Be sure to read the directions carefully for over-the-counter acne treatments; for prescriptions from your doctor, make sure that you are clear as to how much medication you should use, how often you should use it, and how soon you should expect to see results. If you are not sure, call your doctor to review the instructions. It is better to ask twice than to do it wrong.

Some medications, such as Retin-A, should only be used at night because they are inactivated by sun exposure. Others can be used at any time. Some medications must not be combined with others, such as the current formulations of Retin-A and BP, because they may inactivate each other, partially or completely, whereas others work even better when used together, such as topical antibiotics and BP.

40. Why are there so many different treatments for acne?

In a nutshell, so many treatments are available for acne because no one treatment is perfect and because there are so many underlying reasons, both internal and external, that either cause acne directly or at least cause acne to flare in an individual. For this reason, there is, by definition, the need for several different approaches. Also, if you look at the treatments available, there are lots of variations on similar themes. Medications are combined and delivered in a variety of ways to make them more appealing and effective and to increase your likelihood of using them on a regular basis. Also, the skin can adapt to any particular treatment, as can the bacteria that is responsible for certain types of acne, which means that we often have to rotate treatments in order to maintain clearance. Topical treatments are the mainstay of acne treatments. They are used alone or in combination with oral medications to treat and control acne breakouts.

Because many of these treatments have different modes of action, they are often used together in various combinations for maximal benefit in the treatment of acne. Combination treatment is now the standard of care in acne therapy. The newest drugs coming to the market are focusing very highly on creating prepackaged combinations to help increase compliance and simplify acne treatment regimens.

41. Is there a difference between creams, gels, ointments, lotions, or foam formulations in any given topical medication?

Vehicle

the part of the product that holds the active ingredient, e.g., an oil, gel, or cream base into which the medication is added.

The **vehicle** is part of the product that holds the active ingredient. It is the base, or the part of the product that gives it substance. It plays a critical role in how well the active ingredients are absorbed and tolerated. In some cases, the active ingredient can be made much stronger or weaker, depending on its vehicle. In the end, the vehicle is often as important as the active ingredients in achieving satisfactory treatment results from topical acne therapies.

There is an old saying in dermatology: "If it is wet, dry it. If it is dry, wet it." This is true for the vehicle. When the skin is very oily, gels are much better tolerated. When the skin is very dry, products that come in creams or ointments are more appropriate. Lotions and oils are usually better used in the summer months or when there is more humidity in the air.

The more moisturizing a product, the greasier it is, making it unacceptable to most people. On the other hand, the more drying a product is, the more irritating it can be and, again, the less acceptable it is to many people. Sometimes, combinations of more drying and more moisturizing products can be used concomitantly for excellent results. This is true for most acne treatments. Because most topical anti-acne medications are at least somewhat drying, combining them with moisturizers makes them less irritating, which is likely to increase compliance and maximize results.

Another consideration is that some products are more effective when presented in certain vehicles. For example, BP is known to be more active when used in the gel formulation than in the other vehicles that are available; however, it may also be more irritating to some in this formulation, and thus, the options are to use a lower concentration in a gel formulation, to choose a higher concentration in a cream, or to try the cleansers in various strengths.

Topical Acne Treatment

The manufacturers of these medications realize that in order for their products to work, people have to be willing to use them. For this reason, they are constantly working on better and more appealing ways to present their product so that you will keep coming back to their specific brand, even if it costs a bit more. Fortunately, lots of choices are out there already, with more new and improved options becoming available on a regular basis.

42. What is the difference between brand name medications versus the generic options?

Once the patent on any given drug expires, other companies can then apply for approval from the Food and Drug Administration (FDA) for medications using the same active ingredients for the same indications. Getting initial FDA approval can cost millions of dollars and can be very difficult. Once a drug is approved and further tested in the market through use in the general population without further adverse consequences, the company that has the patent on the drug and that went through the trouble to get that approval has a certain amount of time where it is protected from competition.

Once the patent has expired, other companies can bring similar drugs to the market. The amount of testing that they have to do is much less because the active ingredient is already proven. The new product is labeled as a "generic." This makes it a much less expensive venture and is helpful in that it can bring the cost of the medication down significantly.

There are several aspects of a medication besides the active ingredient, however, that affect how well it works and how well it is tolerated in terms of side effects. Sometimes a big difference exists between two drugs that have identical active ingredients. For example, an oral antibiotic can be coated to make it dissolve more slowly, can have fewer side effects, and can be better tolerated when taken with food. The generic may have the same active ingredient, but unless taken on an empty stomach, it may not be absorbed and will therefore not work. Also, it may have an increased side-effect profile in terms of nausea and stomach upset. It may also need to be taken on a different schedule, twice a day or more, for example, instead of once a day for the brand name medication.

For topical medications, the active ingredient is only one part of the equation. Two medications that contain the same quantity or percentage of active ingredient may be much more or less irritating or much more or less effective depending on the other side ingredients in the formulation. It is the vehicle in which the active ingredient is framed that allows for the medication to be absorbed into the skin and exert its effect.

Studies show that some of the generics, which have the exact same active ingredients, are not absorbed into the skin, and the result for the user is increased irritation with decreased efficacy. This is not true for all medications, but it is not rare either. There may also be a difference in the preservatives and fragrance used in one formulation as opposed to another. These can make a difference in how well you tolerate the product being used.

For this reason, it is important to review with your doctor whether it matters for any given prescription if it is filled as brand name or generic at the pharmacy, and then make sure that you get exactly what your doctor prescribed to ensure that you get the best results from your treatment.

43. When I start my treatment, will my acne get worse before it gets better?

Depending on the medication used, there can be an adjustment period where the skin adapts to the treatment. In the process, the skin can look red and feel irritated or more sensitive, and there can be scaling of the skin, which feels like layers of the skin are peeling off. This can be minimized by increasing moisturizing of the area and by starting more slowly.

I usually recommend starting only one new medication at a time when possible so that if there is an unacceptable reaction it will be more clear as to which is the most likely offending agent. Also, you can usually start by using the medication less often and then increasing as your skin tolerates it. Also, most people use too much of the product at one time. You only need to use just enough to get a thin coat over the skin; anything else is only waste and increases the risk of irritation.

What people often perceive as their skin getting worse when they start a new treatment is simply irritation and peeling from this adjustment. If the predominant type of acne is comedonal and the comedones are deep under the skin, sometimes the skin may look temporarily worse as these lesions move through to the surface and are expelled. This can take 1 month or longer to run its course.

44. Can I continue topical or oral treatments while I am pregnant? How long should I wait before I get pregnant?

Because acne often seems to be at its worst when women are at the height of their child-bearing potential, it is very important to let your doctor know all of the medications that you are using to treat your acne, even the over-the-counter medications, if you become pregnant. In most cases, your doctor will simply tell you to stop therapy, at least for a while.

There are questions about using topical retinoids during pregnancy. There are natural levels of isotretinoin and retinoic acid in the blood even in people who have never been exposed to topical retinoids. If you put Retin-A on the skin, the blood level of retinoic acid does not change. Your body eliminates more retinoic acid, but the blood level stays the same. I still believe that the smartest course is not to use retinoids during pregnancy because even the theoretical risk of a problem is not worth it; however, generally, most dermatologists agree that it is okay to stop using the retinoid once you think you may be pregnant.

The one instance in which there is a very real and serious concern regarding acne medications and pregnancy is if a pregnant woman was taking oral isotretinoin (Accutane, Sotret, others) either while pregnant or if she becomes pregnant within 1 month of taking the drug. This medication must not under any circumstances be taken during pregnancy, and women taking oral isotretinoin must discontinue the drug at least 4 weeks before even trying to get pregnant. It is so important that women who plan to take isotretinoin must have adequate contraception to ensure that they will not get pregnant either during the treatment or for 4 weeks after. The matter is so important that the various makers of oral isotretinoin instituted programs called System to Monitor Accutane-related Teratogenicity (S.M.A.R.T.), or variations of it, to help ensure that women do not get pregnant while taking this medication or for at least 1 month after. These programs offer in-depth booklets and videos to help explain the risks of getting pregnant during this time and the methods available to avoid pregnancy.

Some of the birth defects that are associated with oral isotretinoin are as follows:

- Skull abnormalities/deformities
- Ear abnormalities/deformities
- Deafness
- Cleft palate
- Brain abnormalities/deformities
- Heart abnormalities/deformities
- Hormonal abnormalities

Erythromycin

an antibiotic commonly used to treat skin infections.

Azelaic acid

a natural material produced by a yeast that is used as a topical treatment for mild to moderate acne.

In many countries, topical BP and topical **erythromycin** can be used during pregnancy although BP is in the pregnancy category C. **Azelaic acid** is also approved for use by pregnant women in some countries, and is rated pregnancy category B. Topical retinoids are not recommended for use in pregnant women.

For pregnant women who have severe acne or acne that leaves significant scars, oral tetracyclines, including doxycycline and minocycline, are not only *not* recommended, they are **contraindicated**—that is, the prescribing doctor should not offer them at all because they are harmful to the developing fetus. This puts them in the pregnancy category D. Oral trimethoprim is also not recommended.

Contraindicated
a medication or procedure that should not be provided to or performed upon a patient with a particular illness because it will cause harm.

Erythromycin is considered the safest choice, followed by topical azelaic acid. It is important to review with the obstetrician before any medication for acne is used. The obstetrician may tell you to hold off on certain treatments until after the first trimester of pregnancy.

The FDA's system divides drugs into five categories, ranging from completely safe to absolutely forbidden in pregnancy. To qualify for a particular category, a drug must pass (or fail) certain scientific tests in animals, humans, or both. The exact standards for each category are shown in Table 11.

Except for "A" and "X", you can see that these ratings do require a judgment call. Harm to the baby is never a certainty, and some drugs, such as epilepsy medications, may be so crucial to the *mother's* safety as to make taking them the least risky choice.

If a drug is rated "X," there's no question: Avoid it at all costs if you even *think* you're pregnant. But generally if it falls into the "B" or "C" categories, check with your doctor before discontinuing it. Its risks may be low enough, and its benefits sufficiently high, to make its continued use the wisest course.

Table 11. Pregnancy Categories

Category A	Generally considered safe

Controlled studies show no risk in first trimester
No evidence of second- or third-trimester risk
Risk of fetal harm remote

Category B	Caution advised

Animal studies show no risk or adverse fetal effects but controlled human first-trimester studies are not available
No evidence of second- or third-trimester fetal risk
Fetal harm possible but not likely

Category C	Weigh risk/benefit

Animal studies show adverse fetal effect, but no controlled human studies or no animal or human studies are available

Category D	Weigh risk/benefit

Positive evidence of human fetal risk
Maternal benefit may outweigh fetal risk in serious or life-threatening situations

Category X	Contraindicated

Positive evidence of serious fetal abnormalities in animals, humans, or both
Fetal risk clearly outweighs any maternal benefit

45. I used topical Neosporin, bacitracin, or triple antibiotic cream to clear my acne, but it didn't help at all. Why?

These topical antibiotic preparations are very effective against specific types of bacterial infections that are common to the skin, such as staphylococcus or streptococcus skin infections. They are, however, not effective against *P. acnes*. In fact, the ointment can even be occlusive, which can make the acne worse. The medications designed to treat acne are, likewise, ineffective against many of the other bacteria that can cause different types of skin infections other than acne.

When looking for topical treatments for acne, look for labels that indicate that the medication is designed specifically for the treatment of acne and not just for general infections of the skin.

46. Should I moisturize my face while I do these treatments?

Some consider the use of moisturizers in people with acne to be controversial. Moisturizers are not required; however, they can make acne treatments much more tolerable and can improve the quality of skin that may be overly dry from the acne treatments. I am of the school of thought that says the treatment should not be worse than the condition. If your skin is overly dry and irritated from the medicines, then you will likely be unhappy and less compliant with the treatment. Moisturizers can help minimize the sometimes overwhelming dryness that can occur from otherwise very effective acne therapy. If the excessive dryness persists, a change in the medications may be indicated.

If your skin is very oily, moisturizers are not required and need not be used. The best time to use a moisturizer is when your skin feels dry or if you know that you are prone to having easily irritated skin. It is also helpful to use moisturizers alone with the retinoid category of acne medications, either mixed with the retinoid or applied right over it, especially when first starting treatment, in order to minimize the irritation and peeling that may otherwise occur.

Many moisturizers are available, the vast majority of which are over the counter. In choosing a moisturizer that is right for you, look for one that is designed specifically for the face, if this is the area that needs moisture, and look for one that has an SPF of 15 or higher if you are using it in the morning. In this way you can address two important issues at once: You can moisturize your skin, and you can protect it from the damaging rays of the sun, the effects of which may be magnified by the acne regimen that you are on. Look for moisturizers with "nonacnegenic" or "noncomedogenic" written on the label or packaging.

Finding the right moisturizer can be an ordeal of trial and error. I usually recommend that people use a moisturizer that is more rich and creamy at night because there is greater water loss from the skin at night and a lighter cream or lotion in the morning, with an SPF, of course. The moisturizer is applied over the morning acne regimen, and any makeup can be applied over the moisturizer, as desired. Step one would be to wash/exfoliate; step two would be to use a toner, if you are so inclined. Step three is to use the topical medication, followed by the final step of moisturizer with or without sunscreen depending on the time of day.

47. Is benzoyl peroxide (BP) safe?

Benzoyl peroxide (BP) is a staple of acne treatment in the United States. It is generally considered to be safe and effective product for treating acne. It is available in a variety of formulations and concentrations, ranging from 1% to 10%. The gel formulations are generally more stable and are preferable to the creams and lotions. They also allow for a more consistent release of the active ingredient.

BP cleansers are useful for application to large areas such as the chest and back and can be used conveniently in the shower.

In general, people with skin that tends more toward dry should start with lower concentrations of BP products, especially on the face. As with all topical medications, the product should be applied to the entire affected area, usually in the morning and evening, and not only to the visible lesions.

BP offers good efficacy against superficial inflammatory lesions since it has the ability to rapidly suppress the *P. acnes* present in the skin. BP also has the advantage of not being associated with antimicrobial resistance. For this reason, it is often used in combination with other oral or topical antibiotics to increase efficacy and minimize resistance. It has been shown that BP in combination with topical erythromycin or **clindamycin** is more effective and better tolerated than either BP or the topical antibiotic alone.

Clindamycin
an antibiotic effective against specific bacteria, sometimes used in acne treatment.

The main limitation of BP for some acne patients is concentration-dependent stinging, irritation of the skin, contact dermatitis, dryness, and bleaching fabric or hair it comes in contact with. The irritant/contact reaction in the skin is seen as redness, scaling and itching, or burning. These side effects usually occur within the first days to weeks of treatment and improve with continued use of the product. BP is known to bleach hair, clothes, and bed linens that it comes in contact with, and this must be taken into consideration as a risk when this treatment is considered.

BP also works exceptionally well when used in combination with a topical retinoid. In this case, it is probably best to use the retinoid in the evening and BP or a topical antibiotic or combination of BP/topical antibiotic in the morning because this will minimize the risk of inactivation of the retinoid. Also, it is a good idea to put clothing on first, especially if they are to pass over the face in order to minimize contact and the possible bleaching of the fabric that may ensue. Newer formulations are being developed, and further testing is being done to show that these products can be used simultaneously without increased irritant reaction or inactivation of any of the active ingredients (Table 12).

Table 12. Benzoyl Peroxide Formulations

Brevoxyl	4.8% creamy wash; 4.8% gel
Benzac AC	2.5%, 5%, 10% gel (emollient, water base)
Benzagel	5%, 10% (alcohol base)
Benzashave	5%, 10% shaving cream
Desquam-E	2.5%, 5%, 10% gel (emollient, water base)
Triaz wash, pads, gel	3%, 6%, 9%
BenzaClin	1% clindamycin/5% BP gel (water base)
Benzamycin	3% erythromycin/5% BP gel (alcohol base)
Zoderm	4.5%, 8.5% in urea base

48. What topical antibiotics are available?

Topical antibiotics are a mainstay of doctor-prescribed acne therapy. They are uncommonly used as monotherapy because resistance to the medications would become a problem for most people.

The two main topical antibiotics used in acne are erythromycin and clindamycin. These are formulated alone or in combination with BP. They come in solutions, gels, creams, lotions, and wipes. They are also used in combination with zinc. They come in a variety of vehicles such as water, alcohol, oil-free, or oil-in-water mixtures. A very large variety of formulations of these products make them appealing to all skin types, from the oiliest to the most sensitive. Side effects are mostly caused by the vehicle and include stinging, burning, dryness, contact dermatitis, peeling, itching, and redness. These can be minimized by using a formulation that works best for your skin and using only as much of the product as is needed to cover the acne, not the entire tube or jar at a time.

No over-the-counter products contain erythromycin or clindamycin. The over-the-counter products generally contain BP, sulfa-based medications, or salicylic or hydroxy acid, in various strengths. There are also many creative tinted formulations that help conceal the acne while treating it (Table 13).

49. Are retinoids right for me?

The term "retinoid" includes both naturally occurring and synthetic products that classically were related to vitamin A (retinol). However, the newer classification describes retinoids as products that elicit specific

Table 13. Topical Antibiotic Formulations

Akne-mycin	2% Erythromycin ointment or 2% solution
BenzaClin	1% Clindamycin, 5% BP gel (water base)
Benzamycin	3% Erythromycin, 5% BP gel (alcohol base)
Cleocin T	1% Clindamycin solution/50% alcohol 1% Clindamycin gel 1% Clindamycin lotion (oil free) 1% Clindamycin pledgets/50% alcohol
Clindets	1% Clindamycin pledgets/50% alcohol
Emgel	2% Erythromycin gel
Erycette	2% Erythromycin pledgets/66% alcohol
Eryderm	2% Erythromycin solution/77% alcohol
Erygel	2% Erythromycin gel/92% alcohol
Erymax	2% Erythromycin solution/66% alcohol
Staticin	1.5% Erythromycin solution
Theramycin	2% Erythromycin solution/86% alcohol (zinc acetate base)
Topicycline	Tetracycline solution
T-stat	2% Erythromycin solution/86% alcohol 2% Erythromycin swabs
Azelex	20% Azelaic acid cream (oil free)
Finacea	15% Azelaic acid cream

responses by acting at specific sites called retinoid receptors. There are several different retinoid receptors in the skin.

Before topical tretinoin became available in 1971, no other form of acne therapy was available that showed significant improvement in comedones. As a result, topical tretinoin revolutionized acne therapy. The limiting factor of tretinoin was that in the original formulations it was very irritating to the skin. Since then, our understanding of how tretinoins work has grown, and many new formulations have been developed that minimize irritation while maintaining efficacy. Even now, topical retinoids produce the greatest impact in the improvement of acne. We are also continuing to learn about the effects of retinoids on different types of acne as well as on aging skin every year. It has also been shown that tretinoin works for both comedonal and inflammatory types of acne. For these reasons, Tretinoin and tretinoin-like medications have become the mainstay of most acne therapies, effective when used either alone or in combination with other topical or oral treatments. Some of these preparations are less irritating than others, with studies showing that Adapalene (Differin) is the least irritating of the group (Table 14).

50. What do retinoids do for my skin?

The wonderful part about retinoids is that they affect several of the most important steps in the path to acne formation. They get to the root problem of acne by preventing microcomedo formation. They decrease the number of existing comedones and block pathways that lead to inflammation. Several studies have shown

Table 14. Retinoids

1. Tretinoin
Retin-A	0.025%, 0.05%, 0.1%—all available in cream, gel, and solution
Retin-A micro	0.04%, 0.1%
Renova cream	0.02%, 0.05%
Avita	0.025% cream or gel
Generic tretinoin	0.025%, 0.05%, 0.1%
2. Adapalene
Differin	0.1% cream (oil free), gel, pledgets, and solution
3. Tazarotene
Tazorac	0.5% cream (oil in water), gel
	0.1% cream (oil in water), gel

that there is an enhanced therapeutic benefit when topical retinoids are used along with other topical and oral treatments for acne. Irritation from retinoids is still an issue in that some people are very sensitive to these treatments; however, patient education and proper use reduce this potential side effect.

Erica's comments:

I started using Tazorac (tazarotene) every other night, but my skin got very red and started to peel within a week, especially on my chin. I had to stop using it for a while, and I added a face moisturizer. That really helped. I finally got the hang of it, and my skin adjusted to the medicine with really great results. My pimples finally started clearing after about 1 month of using the medicine, along with my benzoyl peroxide face wash, and I am really happy with the results, except for a few pimples around my period. My next problem was that I had a vacation planned, and I was afraid to keep using the medicines because I heard that I would be more likely to get a sunburn. I stopped everything for my vacation, but when I got back, it was like starting all over again with getting my skin used to the treatment. It seemed like a lot of work.

I usually recommend that retinoids be initially used every other day or even only once or twice a week to help the skin adapt to the treatment. Depending on how the skin responds, the applications can increase to every other night and then increase slowly to every night as the skin adapts to the medication. It is important to apply the retinoid at night because the sun inactivates the retinoid. Retinoids are not photosensitizers. This means that they do not increase your sensitivity to sun exposure. They do help your stem cells mature in a more normal way, which can—at least early on—make your skin more sensitive to the sun.

Retinoids are commonly used in climates that are constantly sunny, such as California, Arizona, and Florida. I do not recommend stopping the treatment for those planning vacations to sunny climates.

I simply recommend that they be more vigilant about applying sunscreen and other sun protective behavior, such as wearing a hat and trying not to be out in the middle of the day when the sun is at its peak. Remember the shadow rule: The shorter your shadow, the more dangerous the rays of the sun—at noon, the sun is at its peak and you have no shadow. Try to stay in the shade or indoors during this time if possible, even if you are not using a retinoid.

51. Can I have my lip/face waxed while I am using Retin-A?

It is recommended that you stop the Retin-A for about 5 to 7 days before and 2 days after having lips, brows, or face waxed in order to minimize irritation and "burning" from the procedure. Even if the retinoid is being applied to only the forehead and cheeks, the skin on the upper lip can still be more sensitive to waxing or other potentially irritating procedures. Other areas of the body that are not being treated with Retin-A are not affected. Legs and bikini or other areas not being treated with the retinoid can undergo waxing procedures as usual.

52. Can I use topical treatments while I am taking oral medication?

The effectiveness of oral medications is increased and complimented when used in conjunction with topical treatments. Most commonly a BP cleanser or gel is initially used, followed by a retinoid and/or azelaic acid. Once the acne is under control and you are ready to stop the oral antibiotics, a topical antibiotic can be added to complete the treatment regimen.

53. Can I use topical antibiotics or BP while I am pregnant?

Some of these agents are acceptable for use in pregnancy. It is important to consult with your obstetrician regarding all medications that you are using, including both prescription and over-the-counter medications. Different drugs are rated and categorized into pregnancy categories. The most important pregnancy category to be aware of is category X, which means that the medication is absolutely contraindicated in pregnancy. Accutane (see Question 66) is one medication that falls in to this category. Tetracycline is rated pregnancy category D, which means that it is known to be unsafe for use in pregnancy. Erythromycin is considered to be pregnancy category B, which is generally considered safe in pregnancy. My personal feeling is that you should not take or use any medications during pregnancy that you don't absolutely have to (see Question 44 and Table 11).

54. What is steroid acne?

Corticosteroids, such as oral prednisone, are the gold standard for anti-inflammatory medications. Strong topical corticosteroids are limited by the potential for delayed side effects, including thinning of the skin, stretch marks, new blood vessel formation in the skin (commonly called broken blood vessels), papulopustular flares of acne, and skin addiction to the steroid so that when it is withdrawn there is a rebound flare of the acne.

When topical or oral steroids are used in high enough doses over long periods of time, adverse effects exist that go beyond the skin, such as the risk of developing **cataracts** and suppression of the body's own production of cortisols under periods of stress, which can be very serious; however, a short course (5 days to 2 weeks) may be useful as part of the initial strategy in treating severe inflammatory acne.

One of the main benefits of this approach is to kick start the improvement and get quick control of the situation. Oral steroids may be preferable in very severe inflammatory acne because a short course will immediately reduce the number of inflammatory lesions. As with topical steroids, this can have a significant positive psychologic effect. In addition, the reduction in the severe cystic lesions reduces the pain and/or itching associated with them. When oral steroids are used,

Corticosteroids

a group of anti-inflammatory drugs often used to inhibit allergic reactions or to treat severe inflammation.

Cataract

an opacity in the eye that obstructs vision. Cataracts are usually caused by UV exposure, diseases such as diabetes, or simple aging.

they are most commonly given along with oral antibiotics or isotretinoin. If oral steroids are recommended, your doctor will review with you the potential side effects. It is important to understand that this class of steroids, called glucocorticoids, is very different from the anabolic steroids sometimes used by athletes and body builders.

An injection of the steroid called cortisone in various concentrations directly into inflammatory lesions is a mainstay of acne treatments. It can be especially helpful for large inflammatory lesions. There is a slight risk of localized thinning of the skin, which may or may not resolve within a few months. The treatment is best done early on in the inflammatory process to both minimize the inflammation and clear the lesion more quickly. Other acne treatments can be continued without interruption.

Injections can be especially useful for the occasional flare of inflammatory acne or the few lesions that often come with monthly menstrual periods in an otherwise successful acne management routine; however, if you find that you are going in weekly for injections, then you probably need to reconsider your overall acne regimen.

55. Why does my treatment stop working after a while?

Because acne is a chronic condition of the skin that can wax and wane over a period of many years, treatments occasionally need to be adjusted in order to account for flares of the acne or acne that becomes resistant to the current treatment.

Most acne treatment regimens are done on a rotational basis, meaning that you start with one regimen that works for you. Over time, you many notice that in spite of using the products as directed, you start to get new lesions on a regular basis. One or all of the medications will then need to be changed. When the new regimen again becomes less effective, the rotation continues to either new products or products that were effective in the past but have not been used for a while.

John's comments:

I was doing great on my treatment for a while; I was taking an oral antibiotic and using Retin-A. Then I noticed that I started to get new pimples that just wouldn't go away. I was good about taking my medicine on time and using the cream every night. It seemed as if my skin just decided to ignore the treatment. It was very frustrating to feel like I was doing everything right but was still breaking out.

If oral antibiotics are taken indefinitely, resistance to the medication can occur. It is helpful to limit the time that oral antibiotics are taken to 3 to 4 months at a time followed by a rest period. It is also very helpful to use a topical BP in order to minimize resistance to the topical or oral antibiotics. It is not usually recommended to use an oral antibiotic and a dissimilar topical antibiotic at the same time. Retinoids are very useful in conjunction with oral antibiotics or other regimens but can increase irritancy or skin sensitivity, especially in the first few weeks of treatment.

John's comments:

When I first started the treatment, I tried using a topical BP gel twice a day, but my skin got very irritated and red and kept peeling off. Because I was doing so well just taking a pill every day and using the Retin-A, I stopped using the topical BP. I guess it made a difference in the end.

Oral antibiotics may be used to get quick control of the acne. They should be used in conjunction with topical medications so that when the oral antibiotics are discontinued the topical medications continue to maintain clearance. Starting with an oral antibiotic also allows for the topical medications to be applied on an incremental scale so that the skin has time to adapt to them.

If the BP is too irritating, you can start with a BP cleanser once a day or every other day and then increase slowly to once or twice a day. BP cleansers are also helpful for affected areas of the body other than the face because BP is known to bleach clothing and bedding, which can be disconcerting and expensive when you have to buy new shirts and sheets.

If using topical BP creams or gels, you may want to use a lower concentration and to start by using them once a day or every other day and slowly build up. It is also helpful to look for formulations that are water based rather than alcohol based because alcohol-based mixtures are definitely more drying. Another helpful hint is to apply a moisturizer over the topical medication. Look for moisturizers that are noncomedogenic, and if using them in the morning, look for moisturizers that also have an SPF of at least 15. Many products are available to choose from—so many, in fact, that it can be overwhelming. Try using richer formulations at night and lighter ones in the morning.

John's comments:

I stopped taking the oral antibiotics. I was switched to a BP wash, a topical antibiotic in the morning while continuing the Retin-A at night. My skin got a little red and peely at first, so I backed off the Retin-A for a few days and used a face lotion in the morning. Then I added back the Retin-A every other night for a week, and then I used it every night again. Every so often my skin gets irritated, so I take a day or two off from the Retin-A; that really seems to help. The times that I have the most problems are when I have exams or a big event coming up. I really like that I have control over when I use my medications. At first it was confusing, but eventually I got into my own routine. I know that if I am playing sports or going to the gym more, my acne is going to need more attention; I take the BP wash to the gym and use it right after I work out. My biggest problem is that when I get home at night I am really tired so I don't feel like paying attention to my skin. In the morning, I am always in such a hurry that I sometimes don't get a chance to use the creams.

I often recommend that treatments be adjusted as needed so that they are used more often when the skin feels oilier or around times that are known to cause flares of acne for any given patient. On the other side, I recommend that treatments be adjusted downward when needed as well, to every other day or less, depending on the medications being used, or to increase moisturizing in order to minimize dryness and irritation. Also, some of the medications come in individually wrapped wipes and can be carried to school or work and used when needed during the day for those who are too busy or too rushed first thing in the morning.

There are many variations of product delivery to accommodate even the busiest or laziest user. The idea is to maximize compliance with any given treatment regimen and to improve the results.

PART FIVE

Oral Antibiotics

When should I consider taking oral antibiotics?

If I take an oral antibiotic, will it make me resistant to antibiotics if I really need to take them at a later time?

What are the most common side effects of oral antibiotics?

More ...

56. When should I consider taking oral antibiotics?

The choice between topical and systemic medications is generally based on the presence, extent, and severity of inflammatory lesions. For best results, antimicrobial agents should be combined with topical retinoids and a topical BP product. This increases efficacy, shortens the treatment duration, and helps prevent antibiotic resistance.

In the new age of acne treatment, combination therapy is generally the rule. This means that you should be on more one type of medication at any given time. Because BP is so effective at minimizing resistance to *P. acnes*, it helps maintain the effectiveness of both oral and topical antibiotics and should be used along with them unless there is an allergy to BP. In those cases, BP is not an option, and other treatments are used.

The main indication for oral antibiotics is moderate to severe inflammatory acne. Tetracyclines are the most commonly used family of antibiotics along with a class of antibiotics known as macrolides, and a third class called sulfonamides. Topical antibiotics and BP are indicated in people with mild to moderate inflammatory acne. It is highly recommended that topical treatments, such as with BP and azelaic acid or retinoids, be used in combination with oral antibiotics in order to speed the treatment results and to minimize the resistance of the bacteria to the antibiotic.

Oral antibiotics work by reducing the number of *P. acnes* and *Staphylococcus epidermidis* in the skin. *P. acnes* is thought to trigger the inflammatory response in acne and therefore plays an important role in the formation of acne lesions. Also, antibiotics have an anti-

Table 15. Oral Antibiotics Commonly Used for Acne

- Tetracyclines
  - Tetracycline (generic)
  - Lymecycline
  - Doxycycline
    - Periostat
    - Doryx
  - Minocycline
    - Dynacin
- Macrolides
  - Erythromycin
  - Clindamycin
  - Azithromycin
- Sulfonamides
  - Trimethoprim/sulfamethoxazole (Bactrim)
- Cotrimoxazole

inflammatory activity, which makes them especially useful in inflammatory acne treatment (Table 15).

When taking an oral antibiotic, it is important to know the dose you are taking and how many times a day you should take the medicine. Also, it is generally not a good idea to take these medications right before bedtime because this can lead to an irritation of the esophagus.

Elanor's comments:

I was working on a very big case that was going to trial, and there was no way I was going to court with a face full of pimples. I was started on an oral antibiotics, but I didn't get the medicine for a few weeks because I had to mail in the prescription. I never read directions on these things, after all, how hard could it be, and I knew I only had to take one pill a day. I could do that. The problem is that I often did not get home until well after midnight. One evening, I got home especially late. Just before I crashed, I swallowed my antibiotic pill without water.

I woke up 2 hours later with the most excruciating chest pain. The pain radiated down my left arm. I was sure that I was having a heart attack, so I went to the local emergency room. I told them the medicines I was taking, but they didn't think that was relevant. They gave me morphine and did a lot of tests to see if I was having a heart attack. I am only 27, but I guess it could happen. I felt awful. As it turned out, I didn't have a heart attack at all. The whole problem was that I took the medicine before going to bed, without any water, and I got what my doctor tells me is an irritation of my esophagus. It can feel exactly like a heart attack. I definitely learned to never take anything before bed unless it very clearly says to and to always take my pills one at a time with a full glass of water.

Esophagitis

inflammation of the esophagus.

Esophagitis, or inflammation of the esophagus, which is the connection from the mouth to the stomach, can occur from oral antibiotics, other medications, or even food taken or eaten too soon before bedtime, with some oral antibiotics being more at risk for causing this than others. It is most commonly reversible, and stopping the medicine is often curative. It does serve as a strong reminder to take medications only as directed and to not share your medicines with friends or family. Be sure to tell your doctor about any side effects that you may be having, as the medication may need to be adjusted or stopped and changed to a different, more appropriate therapy.

Before considering starting any oral antibiotic therapy, it is very important to review with your doctor any medications to which you are or think you might be allergic. There can be several medications with names that sound very different that may be within the same class or family of drugs and should be avoided if there is an allergy to any of the medications in that family.

Also, some medications should not be taken together. Be sure to review with your doctor and pharmacist all the medications you are taking—including over-the-counter and herbal preparations—so any problems with drug interactions can be avoided.

Oral antibiotics are indicated in cases of moderate to severe inflammatory acne or acne that is not responsive to topical treatments alone. This method of treatment is unlikely to be helpful in comedonal acne without an inflammatory component.

Oral antibiotics are usually given for at least 6 to 8 weeks with a maximum of 12 to 18 weeks. In some cases, however, if other therapies are not tolerated and the oral antibiotics are clearly effective, the antibiotic therapy may be continued indefinitely. If retreatment is necessary, use the same antibiotic that was effective previously; otherwise, an alternative antibiotic may be indicated.

Also, avoid using oral and topical antibiotics at the same time. Oral antibiotics are best used in conjunction with topical BP and topical retinoids. Compliance is essential. Some antibiotics are given once daily, whereas some are indicated twice daily. Some can be taken with food, whereas others should be taken only within a certain amount of time around meals.

57. If I take an oral antibiotic, will it make me resistant to antibiotics if I really need to take them at a later time?

In the ancient days, before the advent of penicillin, simple infections that we now treat within a few days without even needing to miss school or work were often life-threatening events. Resistance to antibiotics is most definitely a big and ever-growing problem in medicine. Resistance means that the medicine no longer works because the bacteria mutate (change) to work around the drug that is trying to kill them. Think of a radar detector and a driver who is bent on speeding without getting caught. The police keep coming out with better radars to catch people who are speeding, and the drivers keep coming out with better radar detectors to avoid the radars that are trying to nab them. We keep coming up with better antibiotics, but if overused or used inappropriately, we give the bacteria a chance to figure out a way to resist the medicine.

Antibiotics are drugs that are used to treat bacterial infections. Many different antibiotics are available because many different types of bacterial organisms can cause different types of infection in different parts of our bodies. *P. acnes* is a type of bacteria that lives only in the follicles of our skin. We use several specific antibiotics to treat this bacterium, and those antibiotics are pretty selective against only that certain type of bacteria. There is no risk of resistance to other types of bacteria that these antibiotics do not cover. When dermatologists worry about resistance of bacterial organisms to antibiotics, they are mostly worried about resistance of the *P. acnes* to the antibiotics that we are currently using to treat it. When you become resistant to one antibiotic it does not mean that you are resistant to other antibiotics. For this reason, dermatologists often rotate the antibiotics they use. Also, after you stop using the drug for a while, the resistance generally goes away and you can effectively use the particular drug again. Different antibiotics also have different side effects, so be sure to review with your doctor the side effects that may occur with the specific medication you are taking so you will know what to do if certain symptoms occur.

There has been a dangerous trend toward taking antibiotics for everything, including viral illness or other symptoms that are clearly not effectively addressed by antibiotics. This increases the likelihood of resistance and puts people at increased risk of infections that are more difficult to treat. Also, compliance is a big issue. If medications are not taken as directed, the chance of the bacteria building resistance against the medication increases and makes that medicine less useful.

As technology has advanced, we have become able to culture infections and determine specific antibiotics to combat the specific threat—analogous to hitting a nail on the head with a hammer rather than with a cannonball. We can divide the different types of antibiotics available into two basic categories: specific and broad spectrum. Bacteria have specific characteristics and personalities.

These traits are well understood scientifically and are very helpful in making drugs against them. Some bacteria, as in the case of *P. acnes*, like conditions in which there is no oxygen and die or become inactive if the oxygen concentration of the environment surrounding them is increased. Some other types of bacteria can survive only if the oxygen concentration is high. There are lots of ways that scientists have been able to classify the different types of bacteria that can infect us and cause problems such as infections of the skin, pneumonia, or other illness.

The specific classes of antibiotics target only some bacteria very well while having no effect on others. This has made treatments more effective in that we know we are targeting what we need, and it minimizes resistance by not exposing us to treatments that we don't need. Broad-spectrum antibiotics target a variety of bacteria and are used in either infections that are more severe or infections that may involve a variety of bacteria. In inflammatory acne, we know that *P. acnes* is the main bacterial culprit. For this reason we can choose antibiotics that specifically target it.

In other types of infections, a variety of organisms could possibly be the cause of the infection. In these cases, we may try to get a sample of the infected area to try to grow out the offending bacteria in the laboratory. Because the person could get very sick while we are waiting for those results, however, we may choose to start the person on a more broad-spectrum antibiotic that would cover the different types of bacteria that we would expect in that type of infection. Once the results of the test come back, we could then change to a more specific antibiotic that would be effective against that particular bacterium, and in this way again help to minimize the risk of resistance in the future.

The antibiotics used in the treatment of acne are a specific class of antibiotics and target a certain group of bacteria and *P. acnes*. Resistance of *P. acnes* to antibiotics is known to occur commonly but is minimized by adding topical BP into the regimen and using the antibiotics for only as long as is needed to gain control of the acne, and then changing to topical antibiotics or maintaining treatment with topical medications. A strong push exists to find stronger selective antibiotics and other medications to treat acne.

Although there are known potential side effects from oral antibiotics and concerns about resistance (which is also an issue mostly in terms of treatment of acne down the road), if the acne is inflammatory and scarring, oral antibiotics can make all the difference. This makes oral antibiotics an excellent treatment choice under certain circumstances. It can help gain control of the acne and minimize scars that might otherwise last a lifetime.

58. Will the antibiotics make my oral contraceptive ineffective?

Oral contraceptives are approximately 99.6% effective. When oral antibiotics are started, the efficacy of the oral contraceptive goes down to about 96%. This improves over the next few months back to about 99%. Physicians and patients need to recognize that the expected oral contraceptive failure rate, regardless of antibiotic use, is at least 1% per year, and it is not yet possible to predict in whom oral contraceptives may fail.

Although some antibiotics are assumed to compromise the effectiveness of oral contraceptives, the question here is whether or not the antibiotics used in the treatment of acne are associated with such a risk. To address this issue, a review was conducted in three U.S. dermatologic practices of the records of 356 patients with a history of combined oral antibiotic/oral contraceptive use who responded to a follow-up questionnaire. There were five pregnancies in 311 woman-years of combined antibiotic/oral contraceptive exposure (a 1.6% annual failure rate) compared with 12 pregnancies in 1245 woman-years of exposure among controls (a 0.96% annual failure rate)—no significant difference.

In addition, there were no significant differences between oral contraceptive failure rates among women who served as both cases and controls or between the two control groups. Side effects potentially linked to reduced oral contraceptive effectiveness (e.g., diarrhea, breakthrough menstrual bleeding) were not reported by the women who became pregnant. It is presumed that individual differences in steroid blood levels are a more important cause of oral contraceptive failure than associated antibiotic therapy. Some doctors recommend that a second form of contraception be used for the few months after oral antibiotics have been taken. This would eliminate the concern, even though the risk is initially very low.

59. What are the most common side effects of oral antibiotics?

The most common side effects of antibiotics include upset stomach and nausea. Other side effects include increased sun sensitivity, headaches, and yeast infections in women. Some antibiotics are more prone to cause some of the side effects than others. For example, sun sensitivity is more of a problem with the doxycycline family of antibiotics; however, the minocyclines have been associated with an autoimmune condition called **lupus erythematosus**, which is usually reversed when the medication is stopped. The erythromycins are known to be more likely to cause stomach upset, even though all antibiotics can cause this. Pseudomembranous colitis is a potentially serious intestinal problem that can uncommonly be caused by any of the antibiotics but is usually associated with clindamycin.

Lupus erythematosus

an autoimmune disorder where antibodies are created against the body's own tissues, leading to a host of symptoms including a rash on the face.

If you get a rash or other symptoms that you think might be due to any medication that you are taking, you should call your doctor immediately for advice. Oral antibiotics should not be combined with isotretinoin because of the potential for a condition called **pseudotumor cerebri**, which feels like a really bad headache (see Question 75). Because most antibiotics are digested by the liver, drinking alcohol should be avoided if possible to limit the stress and potential damage to the liver.

Pseudotumor cerebri

increased pressure build-up on the brain.

60. Can I go in the sun/tanning booth while I am taking oral antibiotics, isotretinoin, or Retin-A?

The types of ultraviolet radiation of concern to skin are ultraviolet A and ultraviolet B (UVA and UVB for short). In natural sunlight, there is 90% UVA and 10% UVB. The majority of reactions from ultraviolet radiation and sun exposure are from UVA, which penetrates through glass and is relatively constant throughout the year.

Tanning booths usually provide approximately 95% UVA and 5% UVB. They often tout increased safety because of the fact that they are lower in concentration of UVB, which is responsible for burning and contributes to skin cancer formation. Research has shown that UVA is responsible for much of what we call photoaging, as it penetrates deeper into the skin and destroys elastic tissue and collagen. It is also a contributor to the development of skin cancer. It also affects the sebaceous glands and encourages them to grow and become more lumpy and prominent in the skin, called **sebaceous hyperplasia**.

Sebaceous hyperplasia

a condition caused by UVA exposure in which sebaceous glands grow and become lumpy and prominent in the skin.

Sebaceous hyperplasia is not a cancerous or precancerous condition but can be unsightly and disconcerting to the sufferer, as there are sometimes many lesions on the face. Also, this type of lesion can mimic a type of

Oral Antibiotics

Basal cell carcinoma

a form of skin cancer affecting the cells at the bottom layer of the skin.

Biopsy

collection of a tissue sample for laboratory examination, usually in cases where cancer or similar disease is suspected.

skin cancer called **basal cell carcinoma**, and a **biopsy** may be required to make a diagnosis of the lesion. Otherwise, there are several ways your doctor can help to minimize the appearance of these otherwise unimportant bumps in the skin.

Besides the fact that you should never use a tanning booth, you should especially avoid tanning salons while you are taking oral antibiotics or isotretinoin or using a retinoid. These products may increase the sensitivity of your skin to sun, each in their own way. Sun exposure is very similar in composition of ultraviolet rays to tanning booths, and thus, excessive sun exposure should be avoided. Sunscreen should be used, even for incidental sun exposure.

61. How long should I be on oral antibiotics?

The usual minimum duration of therapy is 6 to 8 weeks. The maximum duration is usually approximately 12 to 18 weeks. If other therapies are not well tolerated, however, meaning that they are overly irritating to the skin or not effective, and if the oral antibiotic therapy was working well, your dermatologist may rarely opt to recommend that you continue the oral antibiotic indefinitely. This is not an ideal option for most people. Periostat is the newer low-dose oral antibiotic that may be the exception to this general rule. Because the dose is so low, the idea is that it can and should be taken over a long period of time because the incidence of side effects is very low and resistance is not a problem.

After a successful course of antibiotics is completed, you should continue the topical regimen that your doctor prescribed to maintain clearance. Often prescription and over-the-counter treatments can be used together and can complement each other very nicely, but you should let your doctor know about all of the products that you are using on your skin.

Because there is no cure for acne and because so many factors cause the acne to recur, you may still need to retreat with oral antibiotics on occasion if you should have a flare of acne. In that case, your doctor will most likely recommend that you restart the last antibiotic that was effective and again complete a 12- to 18-week course. This pattern may need to be repeated on and off depending on how you do.

62. Will oral antibiotics affect my teeth?

Tetracyclines are deposited in developing teeth, where they then may cause irreversible yellowish brown staining of the teeth. Also, tetracyclines have been shown to inhibit bone growth in developing fetuses. Therefore, tetracycline should not be given to women who are breast feeding or pregnant, especially after the 4th month. It is in the pregnancy category D/X, which means that it is known to be unsafe in pregnancy.

Tetracycline should also not be given to babies or children younger than 8 years of age because staining of the teeth can also be a problem in this age group. The only antibiotic that is considered safe for the treatment of acne in pregnant women or children is erythromycin. These are also usually reserved for cases in which acne is severe or scarring is an issue; otherwise, topical treatments are usually considered the first-line therapy.

63. Can I eat right before/after taking my oral antibiotic?

Several advances have taken place in the realm of antibiotic production. Although the original formulation of tetracycline is still available and is very inexpensive relative to the newer products on the market, it must be taken at least 1 hour before or 2 hours after eating any foods that contain dairy products. Otherwise, it will not be absorbed and will not be effective.

Increasingly, doxycycline and minocycline are being used as alternatives to tetracycline, in cases in which there is no response to tetracycline, or if the person is unable to tolerate tetracycline. These newer antibiotics are derivatives of tetracycline. They appear to be more effective in reducing the *P. acnes* population and reducing inflammation than tetracyclines, and they are less likely to promote drug resistance. The newer formulations are coated so that they are better tolerated and better absorbed, even if taken with food.

Some antibiotics are even better absorbed and are more effective if taken with food, although you should still avoid taking them with iron or calcium supplements. Each drug has its pluses and minuses, and your doctor will select the one that is right for you depending on your concerns and other health issues.

64. Will I be more sensitive to the sun while I am on oral antibiotics?

Most oral antibiotics increase sun sensitivity (some more than others). Doxycycline is known to be associated with increased photosensitivity, and patients should be switched, if possible, to another antibiotic during the summer months or you should be advised to use sunscreen of higher SPF and to reapply it at least every 2 hours, along with wearing a hat when possible. There are newer formulations that can be taken only once a day and have a lower incidence of causing sun sensitivity, although the risk is not eliminated and sun screen should always be used.

The minocycline family is best tolerated in those who cannot avoid sun exposure. It is always recommended that sunscreen of SPF 15 or higher be used and reapplied regularly, meaning at least every 2 hours or more often after bathing or excessive sweating.

65. What other oral therapies are available?

Oral zinc has been shown to be effective against non-inflammatory lesions but does not affect comedones. This is true even in people who do not show signs of zinc deficiency in their blood or skin. Zinc may safely be used in the summer because there is no issue of phototoxicity. It is typically prescribed in a dose of 200 mg/day without food. Side effects at this dose may include upset stomach and nausea. Zinc may be considered as an alternative to tetracyclines, although dermatologists do not commonly use it.

Nicomide is a vitamin supplement that is now available in prescription form to help treat inflammatory acne. It seems to affect the inflammatory types of acne and has had some success when used along with other oral and/or topical medications in the treatment of acne.

Low-dose doxycycline is another form of treatment that is gaining some momentum. When these antibiotics are used at doses much lower than those traditionally considered to be therapeutic, they seem to have at least some effect on the growth of the bacteria. In addition, at these lower doses, there does not seem to be the same adverse side effects or bacterial resistance. They work not by killing off the bacteria, as they would at the higher doses, but by affecting the ability of the bacteria to cause problems in the skin. In the studies done so far, at the end of 6 months, when the low-dose oral antibiotics was used alone, without any other adjunctive treatment, there was a 50% reduction in inflammatory lesions and a 53% reduction in comedones. There was no decrease in the number of *P. acnes* in the skin, nor was the resistance profile affected. The bacteria that were present were simply inactivated. Side effects were minimal to none.

Although the drug's side-effect profile is definitely a plus, six months does, however, seem like a long time to wait for improvement of the acne. The acne was improved, but not completely resolved. The clearance may improve more quickly if combined with topical BP or retinoids. It remains to be determined how useful this drug will be in the long term for the treatment of acne.

PART SIX

Oral Isotretinoin

What is oral isotretinoin?

Am I a good candidate for oral isotretinoin?

How does isotretinoin work?

More ...

66. What is oral isotretinoin?

Isotretinoin is an oral retinoid, meaning that it is in the vitamin A family of compounds. For this reason, many of the side effects that we see from isotretinoin are similar to the effects that we see from taking toxic doses of vitamin A. Isotretinoin is considered an appropriate treatment for people who have severe nodular acne or moderate or severe acne that has not responded to oral antibiotics and topical treatment. Virtually all dermatologists also prescribe oral isotretinoin for moderate to severe acne that scars physically and psychologically, inflammatory acne that does not respond to conventional therapy, and chronic acne that keeps recurring after any given treatment.

With the advent of oral isotretinoin (sold under the trade name of Accutane) and now also as generics (known as Sotret or Amnesty), severe, scarring acne that often left a lifetime of physical and psychologic scars became a much less frequently observed occurrence. Because of the potential for very serious side effects, however, this treatment is not without its perils and is not for everyone. There have been congressional hearings on the drug, and there has been a concerted effort on the part of families whose children have committed suicide while on Accutane and groups that focus on birth defects to try to get this medication off the market.

Roche, which was the original manufacturer of Accutane, along with dermatologists convinced of the need for this very important drug to continue to be available for the treatment of acne, have agreed to specific guidelines and monitoring for patients on oral isotretinoin. This effort has been successful and continues in the form of detailed written consents, written and video information, surveys, and other voluntary registration procedures. The program has been successful in increasing the awareness of the risks of oral isotretinoin while managing to keep it on the market for those who really need it. Over the past 6 months new guidelines have been recommended requiring all patients taking oral isotretinoin to be entered into a formal registry to better monitor those taking the medication.

67. Am I a good candidate for oral isotretinoin?

Oral isotretinoin is the first-line treatment for severe acne and may also be used in people who have failed conventional treatment, such as a combination of topical retinoids, BP, topical or systemic antibiotics, and when appropriate, hormonal therapies (Table 16).

Lily's comments:

I have had acne for over 1 year. At first I just got the regular pimples and blackheads. I tried stuff from the drug store and then oral antibiotics from my doctor. My skin is pretty sensitive, so I use Retin-A every other day and a benzoyl peroxide wash at night. This helped for a while, but now I get painful big bumps under my skin that leave craters when they finally go away. I get a few new ones every month. I also have a lot of regular pimples that make my face look horrible. The oral antibiotics don't work anymore,

Table 16. Consensus Recommendations for Oral Isotretinoin

- Severe nodulocystic acne/severe acne variants
- Inflammatory acne with scarring that has failed conventional treatment
- Moderate-to-severe acne with frequent relapsing
- Acne with severe psychologic distress

and I can't take the scarring. I needed to do something major. I went to my doctor with my parents to talk about oral isotretinoin. The idea of taking a medicine that was so strong and seemed so dangerous was scary, but I really wanted my acne to get better. We talked about the side effects and that the acne could still come back and that I might need to do the treatment again. My doctor gave me a booklet at the end of the visit. I took the booklet home and went over it with my parents. We decided that because my acne was leaving really bad scars and my other treatments stopped working, I would go on the medicine.

68. How does isotretinoin work?

Oral isotretinoin is a retinoid preparation that decreases the size and secretion of the sebaceous glands. It normalizes the skin cells, especially those lining the pores. It prevents the formation of new comedones. It indirectly inhibits the growth of *P. acnes* by changing the environment in which the *P. acnes* usually live, making it much less inviting. It also has an anti-inflammatory effect.

During oral isotretinoin therapy, sebum production is reduced by 90% or more. This leads to a substantial decrease in the levels of *P. acnes*; however, both *P. acnes* and sebum levels increase once the medication is discontinued. This makes oral isotretinoin unique among all of the current oral acne treatments available in that it affects all of the underlying factors behind the process of acne. It makes it a highly effective but sometimes controversial treatment option.

69. Does oral isotretinoin cure acne?

Because acne is an often chronic condition of the skin that is influenced by both genetic and external factors, neither oral nor topical medications can technically cure the condition. Medications can, however, have a profound effect on how active the acne is and how much treatment it can require over time.

At least one third of people who have taken oral isotretinoin will have a relapse of their acne within the first three years after treatment. Because both sebum and *P. acnes* levels increase once oral isotretinoin treatment is complete, acne can recur in some people after an otherwise very effective treatment course. In most cases, oral antibiotics or a second treatment course with isotretinoin can be attempted after a 2-month rest period and, rarely, even a third course if necessary. However, in cases in which there is a recurrence of the acne soon after a treatment course is completed, further evaluation may be helpful in trying to determine whether hormonal influences are a factor, which would then mean that other options should also be considered either instead of or in addition to oral isotretinoin treatment.

70. What dose of isotretinoin is right for me?

The usual dose varies depending on your weight and the severity of your acne. First, you need to determine how much you weigh in kilograms, as opposed to pounds. The dose can range from 0.1 to 2 mg/kg, with the most common dose being 0.8 mg/kg/day divided into two—morning and night. Oral isotretinoin is best absorbed and most effective when taken with food and when taken twice a day.

Your doctor may decide to start you on a lower dose for the first month or two so that you can acclimate to the side effects, to at least some extent, and then increase the dose for the rest of the 16- to 20-week course of therapy. In some cases, higher doses for longer than 20 weeks may be required for adequate results. In some very severe cases of acne, oral **prednisone**, a corticosteroid, is also given for 2 to 6 weeks, usually before oral isotretinoin treatment is begun.

Prednisone
a corticosteroid commonly used to treat inflammation.

Before you start oral isotretinoin, you should have a detailed discussion with your doctor regarding any concerns that you may have about the treatment, and you should be sure to discuss any personal or family history of depression. Your doctor will give you a booklet that the makers of oral isotretinoin provide for you to take home to review and discuss with your family. You will bring this booklet back with you on the next visit because both you and your doctor must sign and date several pages, some of which you will keep, some of which the doctor will keep, and a few of which will be sent to the manufacturer of the drug as part of a survey. At this pre-oral isotretinoin visit, your doctor will also request baseline blood tests, which will be repeated monthly while you are taking the drug.

If you are a woman, your doctor will also review pregnancy and contraceptive issues with you and make sure that you are not pregnant at the start of treatment. It is important to understand that the risk of birth defects exists only while the retinoid is in the body; after the retinoid is cleared, typically 6 weeks after discontinuing therapy, there is no longer a risk. A patient information form and video are available from the manufacturer to help with counseling regarding contraceptive and pregnancy issues (Table 17).

Table 17. Available Doses

Amnesty, Accutane
10-, 20-, or 40-mg capsules that come in 10-packs

Sotret
10-, 20-, 30-, or 40-mg capsules

71. How long is the usual course of oral isotretinoin?

The effect of oral isotretinoin, especially in severe nodulocystic acne, can be dramatic. Most cases of severe acne respond to a single 4- to 6-month treatment course. In general, pustules heal more quickly than papules or nodules. Also, lesions on the face, upper arms, and legs tend to respond more quickly than lesions on the back or chest. In some cases, treatment is started at a low dose in order to help the skin get acclimated to the drug before increasing to a higher dose in the months that follow (Table 18).

72. Will I get worse before I get better? How long will it take before I see results?

In some cases, there can be a flare of the acne in the first month after starting Accutane. There are ways around this. Sometimes a short course of prednisone is given to minimize inflammation and to avoid the flare that would accompany it. In most cases, however, we start at a lower dose and incrementally increase the dose over the first one to two months as the patient acclimates to the drug.

Table 18.   Laboratory Evaluations

Pretreatment evaluation
- Review of side effects
- Review of pregnancy/contraception (women)
- Review of informed consent booklet

Blood tests at pretreatment and weeks 4 and 8
- Baseline fasting cholesterol
- Triglyceride level
- Standard liver function test
- Pregnancy test (women only)

Monthly evaluation
- Review of side effects
- Review of birth control methods
- Physical exam to document improvement
- Answer questions, review results

In general, it takes approximately 1 to 2 months after starting treatment to really see results. This means that there should be fewer or no new lesions, and that the lesions that do come up should be smaller and should resolve more quickly. Results tend to last for at least several months to years after stopping treatment.

73. What are the side effects of oral isotretinoin?

Oral isotretinoin has become a very controversial drug because of some of the side effects associated with it. There have been congressional hearings and several attempts to take this drug off the market. Although some of the side effects can be tragic, close monitoring of patients taking this medication can avoid the worst of the potential adverse reactions. There is no other drug available at this time that can treat and often clear severe, scarring, disfiguring acne. Many have even considered their isotretinoin treatment to be life saving. When there is appropriate counseling and monitoring, oral isotretinoin can really be a miracle cure for many with severe, scarring acne.

Lily's comments:

When I first started taking the medicine, it took a while before I noticed anything. The first thing I felt was that my skin started to feel tight and dry, especially my lips. I was started on a lower dose so that I could adjust to the effects. I didn't really see a change in my acne right away, but at least it didn't get worse. It was also a relief to stop all the other treatments I was using for a while. I was really sick of my routine, especially since it just wasn't working anymore.

Taking one pill twice a day was easy. I was a little concerned about some of the side effects, especially that my hair could fall out and the extreme dryness. I was also not crazy about the idea of having blood tests done every month. I really hate needles.

The second month of treatment was a little easier. I started to see the improvement, and I had a good routine going with my moisturizers. I was careful not to drink alcohol and to use sunscreen every day. I didn't have any headaches or joint aches or hair loss, but I did seem to feel a little achier sometimes, especially if I had a really tough workout.

At every visit my doctor reviewed my blood tests and how I was doing. When I told a few of my friends that I was on Accutane, they all wanted to go on it right away to get rid of their acne too. I liked that they could see the improvement too. I also found that one of my friends had to stop taking it because of a really bad reaction. My friend got very depressed and had to miss school for a while. That scared me a little, but I was feeling fine so I kept going.

Actually, I felt even better than usual since my skin was starting to look so much better. I had more confidence in myself, and I wanted to go out and be with people more. I didn't feel like I had to hide my face like I did before. It isn't that everything was perfect; my face was dry and I still had scars. It's just that I finally had some hope that there might be an end to the acne.

Although the list of potential side effects and adverse reactions from Accutane or the new generic formulation is quite extensive and even overwhelming to many, the most common side effects include dry, chapped lips and dry eyes, dry skin, and dry mouth. Less commonly, there can also be secondary infection with a bacterium called *S. aureus*. This can be treated with topical or oral antibiotics as necessary. Some patients have noted muscle aches and backaches, and some have mild headaches at the start of therapy. Nosebleeds are fairly common, and skin fragility may also occur, especially on the hands.

Any patient with severe headaches, decreased night vision, or signs of adverse psychiatric events should immediately stop taking the drug and call his or her doctor. In addition, serum lipids are usually routinely monitored. This is done by a routine blood test that can be done either at your doctor's office or at a local laboratory test site. Some schools and offices have the ability to do routine blood tests as well.

Oral isotretinoin is a potent teratogen, meaning that it is well known to cause birth defects in children whose mothers get pregnant while taking oral isotretinoin or within 1 month after stopping isotretinoin. For this reason, any woman who is of child-bearing potential who plans on taking isotretinoin must have two negative pregnancy tests before starting treatment and for at least 1 month after therapy. Adequate contraception is essential, and the importance of this cannot be overstated before and during treatment as well as for 4 weeks after discontinuing treatment. Therapy should start on the first, second, or third day of the menstrual period once the results of two negative pregnancy tests have been obtained.

It is important for both the person taking isotretinoin and for their family members to be educated regarding the potential for mood swings and depression during isotretinoin therapy. In most cases, psychosocial events associated with severe acne most often improve once the acne starts to clear; however, in some people with acne who have depression or a tendency toward depression, their psychologic outlook does not improve with the acne treatment. This may be due to several different reasons; however, oral isotretinoin should be discontinued in these cases, and treatment should be instituted for the depression as needed.

Some physicians definitely believe that oral isotretinoin does produce, very occasionally but unpredictably, significant mood changes, depression, and other significant psychiatric side effects. It is very important to discuss these issues with your doctor and to also let your doctor know whether you have been treated in the past for depression or suicide attempts, or whether you have a family history of depression.

Rarely, long-term oral retinoid therapy may be complicated by bone changes, including osteoporosis and other conditions. One study concluded that a loss of bone density occurred as a direct effect of retinoids on bone. Other reports indicate bone changes on oral isotretinoin, such as bone fractures or delayed healing. These are changes that are more typically found in patients on higher doses of the drug than used for the typical acne patient or for those in whom high doses are used over longer periods of time than usual. There are some new formulations of oral isotretinoin that are being tested that are less affected by food and have fewer side effects in terms of dryness of skin, eyes, and mouth and that have less of a potential effect on lipids.

Because oral isotretinoin is metabolized or digested by the liver, as is alcohol, you should try to avoid drinking alcohol while on oral isotretinoin therapy. There have been reports of liver function abnormalities that may have been related to Accutane, most of which improved with either continued administration of the drug or after the medication was stopped. The published reports have been nearly unanimous in showing the lack of isotretinoin-induced liver damage of any kind. However, regular blood tests are still routinely done to ensure normal liver-function values.

Another reported side effect is decreased night vision, which in some cases has lasted even after the treatment was stopped. Finally, there are **parabens** in the Accutane capsule, and thus, people with allergies to parabens should avoid taking oral isotretinoin (Table 19). For a complete list of side effects and potential reactions, consult with your doctor or the company. More information is also available on web sites listed in the Appendix.

Parabens
a group of chemicals used as preservatives in cosmetics, and as antibacterial agents in some antibacterial toothpastes.

Table 19. Potential Side Effects of Oral Isotretinoin

Common
    Dry skin, eyes, and mouth
    Nosebleeds

Uncommon/serious
    Hypertriglyceridemia (liver function abnormalities)
    Headaches
    Mood swings/depression/suicidal ideation
    Pseudotumor cerebri
    Bone changes
    Visual changes

Most serious/avoidable
    Birth defects

74. What should I avoid while taking oral isotretinoin?

Keep this list handy:

- Women should not get pregnant; men should not get a woman on Accutane pregnant while she is taking oral isotretinoin or for at least one month after stopping the drug.
- Use 2 forms of contraceptive (such as oral contraceptive plus a condom) while on oral isotretinoin to make sure pregnancy does not occur.
- Do not breastfeed while taking isotretinoin or for 1 month after stopping.
- Do not give blood while taking isotretinoin or for 1 month after stopping. If someone who is pregnant is exposed to your blood, her baby may be exposed and may have birth defects.

Oral Isotretinoin

131

- Do not take vitamin A supplements; these increase your chances of having side effects.
- Do not have cosmetic procedures to smooth your skin, including waxing or laser procedures, while you are on isotretinoin or for 6 months after you stop.
- Avoid excessive sunlight and ultraviolet lights and tanning booths because this drug can make your skin more sensitive to ultraviolet light.
- Do not use birth control pills that do not contain estrogen (minipills). They may not work while you take Accutane. Ask your doctor to make sure that the pill you are taking is appropriate.
- Tell your doctor if you are taking other drugs or herbal products. Some of these products may decrease the efficacy of the oral contraceptive and would have to be discontinued for the duration of the treatment and for 1 month after.
- Do not share the medicine with other people.
- Do not take isotretinoin with antibiotics unless you talk to your doctor.

75. Can I take antibiotics or use other topical acne medications while I am on oral isotretinoin?

In general, oral isotretinoin is used only as a monotherapy, meaning that once you start oral isotretinoin you should stop all of your other acne treatments. It is well documented that when oral isotretinoin is taken in conjunction with the oral tetracycline class of antibiotics there is an increased incidence in one of the side effects called pseudotumor cerebri. This feels like a really bad, persistent headache, along with nausea, vomiting, and problems with vision. It should be brought to the attention of your doctor immediately. You should also not take vitamin A in high doses while on oral isotretinoin therapy because it is in the same class of compounds, and the combination can increase the risk of toxicity. It is uncommon to prescribe other antiacne medications with oral isotretinoin; however, some dermatologists co-prescribe a nontetracycline antibiotic such as erythromycin for the first month of therapy.

Because most topical acne treatments are at least somewhat drying or irritating, they should be discontinued within 1 month of starting oral isotretinoin treatment. Topical exfoliating agents, Retin-A, and drying agents should be avoided because isotretinoin has a drying effect on the skin and mucous membranes.

It is also helpful to avoid hot showers and drying soaps and to apply moisturizers several times during the day, especially after washing, to prevent dry, chapped skin. People who wear contacts may need to switch to soft lenses or eyeglasses until the dryness resolves.

76. Can I have laser/cosmetic treatments, waxing, or other treatments done while I am on oral isotretinoin?

Because Accutane affects skin cell turnover, it can mean that any surgery or laser resurfacing treatment, or even deeper **chemical peels**, done within 6 months of taking Accutane can lead to excessive scarring and disfigurement. With the advent of the newer lasers available today, known as nonablative lasers because they do not remove the upper layers of the skin, this is probably less of a risk than in the past. Many doctors, however, opt for being more conservative and waiting

Chemical peels
the application of one or more chemicals to the face which 'burn' off damaged cells.

at least 6 months before doing any elective procedure, especially if it is for cosmetic purposes. Laser or intense pulsed light hair removal is sometimes done while on oral isotretinoin, but you should be careful to have the procedure done by a qualified doctor or in a doctor's office, and let the doctor know that you are either still taking or were recently taking oral isotretinoin.

Because the skin is more dry and sensitive while on oral isotretinoin therapy, any treatment that potentially irritates the skin can be a problem. Your skin may react more strongly to waxing or other hair removal methods.

77. How many courses of oral isotretinoin can I take?

Because oral isotretinoin can affect bones and other organ systems, there is a maximal lifetime dose of oral isotretinoin that is considered safe and appropriate in order to minimize the risk of adverse long-term reactions. Most people on a typical course of oral isotretinoin of 0.8 mg/kg for a 16- to 20-week course could do three treatment courses over their lifetime if necessary. Many doctors will use the approximate 0.8 mg/kg as an average treatment dose but will not hesitate to increase the dose in order to get the desired results. Many of the side effects are dose related and can limit the amount of drug given.

Sometimes low-dose oral isotretinoin is very effective in some people, and this not only minimizes side effects but also allows for it to be used intermittently, over time, as needed and with proper monitoring without concern of reaching the maximal dosage.

78. Why didn't oral isotretinoin work for me?

Recurrence of acne is not uncommon after oral isotretinoin treatment. Some people are successfully retreated with oral and topical antibiotics, BP, and topical retinoids, but a significant number require retreatment with isotretinoin. According to one study, only 38% of patients had no acne at the 3-year follow-up after a single course of oral isotretinoin. Among the remaining patients, acne was controlled with topical treatment in some and topical treatment plus oral antibiotics in others, and in a significant number of patients, retreatment with oral isotretinoin was required for adequate results.

The authors of the study noted that relapse was more likely to occur in patients who were 16 years old or younger and in women versus men. Relapse is most common in the first year after treatment. Maintenance treatment with a topical retinoid may reduce the relapse rate.

PART SEVEN

Hormonal Treatments

What is hormonal therapy? Do I need to have my hormones evaluated?

What hormonal therapy is right for me?

Does every oral contraceptive help acne?

More ...

79. What is hormonal therapy? Do I need to have my hormones evaluated?

Hormonal therapy is an excellent option for women, especially if oral contraception is also desired. Hormonal therapy generally implies oral contraceptives, either alone or in conjunction with other hormone treatments. These treatments help women who have acne either alone or in association with other signs of hormonal imbalance such as increased hair growth on the face or other parts of the body where hair growth is undesirable and for women who have excessive hair loss from the scalp unexplained by other factors, such as thyroid or other conditions, and irregular menstrual periods.

The goal of hormonal therapy is to block the effects of androgens on the sebaceous gland and probably the skin cells that are lining the pores as well. This can be accomplished with the use of estrogens or a class of drugs known as antiandrogens (androgen receptor blockers) or by agents designed to reduce the body's production of androgens by the ovary or adrenal gland, such as oral contraceptives, glucocorticoids, or gonadotropin-releasing hormone agonist (Table 20).

Hirsutism

the excessive growth of hair on a woman's face, torso and limbs, and is generally caused by increased androgens. It is a common sign of polycystic ovary syndrome in women.

An evaluation of hormones, usually done by an endocrinologist, may be indicated for women with acne who have proven resistant to conventional treatments or if there is a sudden, severe onset of acne. Other cases in which an endocrine evaluation may be indicated are in women with acne who also have irregular menstrual periods and also increased hair growth in unusual areas such as the face and abdomen (called **hirsutism**). Androgen evaluation may also be indi-

Table 20.   Hormonal Therapy

Antiandrogens
    Cyproterone acetate
    Chlomadinone acetate
    Spironolactone
    Drospirenone
    Desogestrel
    Flutamide

Agents that block androgen production
    Estrogens
    Oral contraceptives
    Cyproterone acetate
    Gonadotropin-releasing hormone agonists
    Low-dose glucocorticoids

cated for women who relapse shortly after oral isotretinoin therapy. The screening usually involves a physical exam by the doctor and a series of blood tests to measure specific levels of hormones in the blood (Table 21).

These screening tests are timed to correlate with a certain phase of the menstrual cycle and are usually done

Table 21.   Hormonal Screening Tests

DHEAS

Total testosterone

Free testosterone

Luteinizing hormone/follicle-stimulating hormone ratio

Prolactin

17-Hydroxyprogesterone

Hormonal Treatments

within 2 weeks before the next menstrual cycle begins. People on oral contraceptive pills should discontinue the medication for at least 1 month before testing. These tests are designed to try to pinpoint the source of the increased androgen production so that appropriate therapy can be instituted.

It is important to note that hormonal therapy can be very effective in women even if the blood levels of the serum androgens are within normal limits. Although women with acne are more likely to have abnormalities in hormonal evaluations than women without acne, most women with acne who are evaluated for hormonal abnormalities have androgen levels that are within normal limits.

Hormonal therapies seem to work best in adult women and sexually active teens with persistent inflammatory papules and nodules that commonly involve the lower face and neck. These women often report that their acne flares before their menstrual periods and consists of painful, often deep, inflammatory papules and nodules. The skin may or may not be oily. There are also often comedones on the forehead and chin, especially in teenagers. These women also note that there is little or no improvement in their acne even after multiple courses of antibiotics.

In these cases, oral antibiotics can be discontinued in favor of oral contraceptives because they block the production of androgens from both the ovary and adrenal glands. Also, the continued use of oral contraceptive pills is recommended if the addition of other hormonal agents is considered for use in the future.

For optimal results from hormonal therapy, appropriate patient selection is key. Hormonal therapy is useful for women with endocrine abnormalities and for women who have proven nonresponsive to or unable to tolerate more conventional therapies such as oral antibiotics, topical antibiotics, and retinoids along with BP. The use of oral contraceptive pills may also be useful for women who require medical treatment to control irregular periods or who would like contraception. It is important to remember that oral contraceptive pills do not protect against sexually transmitted diseases and that a second form of protection is required to reduce the risk of transmission of HIV and other potentially serious sexually transmitted diseases.

The aim of hormonal therapy is to reduce sebum production; however, sebum production is only one component in the pathway to acne. For this reason, hormonal therapy is most effective when used in conjunction with other antiacne therapies, including oral or topical antibiotics, topical retinoids, azelaic acid, salicylic acid, and BP. For those with concerns about the reduced effectiveness of contraception when oral contraceptive pills are used in conjunction with oral antibiotics, recent evidence suggests that antibiotics do not significantly affect the metabolism of oral contraceptive pills, which means that their effectiveness in contraception should not be reduced.

The following are recommendations for hormonal therapy:

- It is an excellent choice for women who need oral contraception for gynecologic reasons.
- It should be used early in female patients with moderate to severe acne or signs of androgen abnormalities.

- It is a useful as a component of combination therapy in women with or without documentable hormonal abnormalities.
- It is sometimes used in women with late-onset acne.

80. What hormonal therapy is right for me?

After appropriate evaluation, your doctor will work with you to determine the right medicine or combination of medicines for you.

Estrogen

female sex hormone.

Estrogens are particularly valuable in women who have oily skin and clear signs of increased sebum production. Any estrogen, if given in high enough doses, will decrease sebum production; however, higher doses of estrogen are necessary than that required for typical oral contraception. Estrogens suppress the ovarian production of androgens and encourages the liver to increase the production of a product called sex hormone binding globulin that binds the androgen and takes it out of circulation.

For women on estrogen therapy, breast exams and pap smears should be done at least annually, with the recommendations varying from country to country depending on age, sexual activity, family history of breast and other cancers, and other factors. The incidence of more serious side effects, such as clotting and high blood pressure, that can occur in the use of estrogens is fortunately rare in healthy young women; however, the doctor and the patient should be aware of the potential risk of adverse reactions, and the risk/benefit ratio should be carefully considered before starting estrogen therapy.

Recent data suggest that it is not possible to predict the final effect of an oral contraceptive on sebum production based on the amount or type of estrogen it contains. All of the low-dose estrogens tested showed that sebum production was reduced by about the same amount.

81. Does every oral contraceptive help acne?

Oral contraceptives (OC) should only be used in women over the age of 16 because in younger women they can suppress growth. The main way OC's work to improve acne is by decreasing androgens such as DHEAS and free testosterone, and by increasing sex hormone binding globulin that binds to testosterone and reduces the amount of free testosterone. In this way OC's help inhibit sebum production, which is one of the main components of acne production. The two main active ingredients in most oral contraceptives are estrogens and progestins. Estrogens are known to reduce sebum production, with some types of estrogens being more potent than others. Progestins can increase the androgenic effect, have no effect on it, or decrease it. Some of the progestins increase the effects of androgens directly or can act as antiestrogens, blocking the benefits of the estrogen on reducing sebum production.

Many of the different types of oral contraceptives are effective in the treatment of acne. The only oral contraceptives that can potentially worsen acne are the ones that contain only progestins instead of a combination of progestin and estrogen. Oral contraceptives containing only progestins include levongestrel and medroxyprogesterone. Acne, hirsutism, and hair loss have been associated with certain progestins.

82. What other hormone treatments are available?

Antiandrogens

Cyproterone acetate (CA): This drug blocks the androgen receptor. It is combined with an estrogen called ethinyl estradiol in an oral contraceptive formulation commonly used in Europe for the treatment of acne (Dianette, Diane-35). It is not currently available in the United States. Reports have shown improvement of 75% to 90% in patients taking variations of this medication.

CA works through a dual action of both inhibiting ovulation and blocking the androgen receptors. This drug should be used only in women because of the risk of feminization in men (increased breast size and other effects).

Potential side effects of CA include irregular menstrual periods, breast enlargement, nausea/vomiting, fluid retention (bloating), swelling of the legs, headache, and **melasma**. It can also be associated with tiredness, liver abnormalities, and rarely blood-clotting disorders.

Chlormadinone acetate: Similar to CA, it is available in several European countries and is only slightly less efficacious than CA.

Spironolactone: Spironolactone functions as both an androgen receptor blocker and possibly also an inhibitor of 5-α-reductase type 1. In doses of 50 to 100 mg per day, it has been shown to reduce sebum

Melasma

a skin condition presenting as brown patches on the face of adults.

production and improve acne. In countries such as the United States with no effective antiandrogenic medications such as CA, spironolactone may be used for female patients with therapy-resistant acne, although it has not been formally approved for this condition.

In one study looking at spironolactone therapy in acne, one third of the patients had complete clearing of their acne. One third had marked improvement, and nearly one third showed partial improvement, with less than 10% showing no improvement of their acne.

Side effects are increased at higher doses and include the potential for increased potassium in the blood, a slight lowering of the blood pressure, irregular menstrual periods, breast tenderness and enlargement, headache, and fatigue. The increased potassium in the blood is rare in healthy young women. Although breast tumors have been reported in rats treated with spironolactone, this drug has been used for years in humans and has not been directly linked with the development of cancer. There have been no documented cases of breast cancer in more than 30 years of spironolactone usage.

Because spironolactone is an antiandrogen, there is a risk of feminization of a male fetus if a pregnant woman takes this medication. The risk to a fetus and the symptoms of irregular menstrual periods can be improved by combining the treatment with an oral contraceptive. Side effects can be minimized if treatment is started at a low dose of 25 mg per day and increased every few months as needed because the response can take as long as 3 months, as with other hormonal therapies. Once adequate response is attained, dosage can again be lowered to the minimal dose required to maintain adequate results.

Flutamide: Flutamide blocks the androgen receptor and is approved for the treatment of prostate cancer. It has been used at doses of 250 mg twice a day in combination with oral contraceptives for the treatment of acne or hirsutism in women. In a study comparing Flutamide with spironolactone, Flutamide was shown to be superior in reducing total acne after just 3 months.

Side effects can be serious, including cases of fatal **hepatitis**, requiring regular blood tests to monitor liver function. As with all antiandrogens, pregnancy should be avoided because of the risk of feminization in male fetuses. The use of Flutamide in acne is very much limited by the side-effect profile and is used very little.

Oral contraceptive pill: These drugs work by blocking ovarian androgens. They contain estrogens, often in conjunction with progestins, to avoid the risk of **endometrial cancer** associated with the use of estrogens alone. Some progestins also have their own androgenic potential, which can aggravate the acne.

Several generations of progestins are now available, the most recent of which has the lowest intrinsic androgenic activity. Many oral contraceptives are available that offer a variety of types, combinations, and dosages of estrogens and progestins. This means that for most women at least one oral contraceptive will have some effect on their acne while also offering contraception. For a woman who is considering starting an oral contraceptive as a form of birth control, she should also bring up any issues of acne in order to maximize the

Hepatitis

any disease featuring inflammation of the liver. Hepatitis can be caused by viral infection, alcohol or drug abuse, or exposure to certain toxins.

Endometrial cancer

the most common type of uterine cancer.

benefits of the drug. She should at least make sure that the oral contraceptive pill that she is considering would not potentially make her acne worse.

All combination oral contraceptive pills reduce the amount of free testosterone circulating in the blood and have had a positive effect on acne in laboratory tests, although this has for some reason not always translated to improved acne in people.

The most serious side effect of oral contraceptive pills is **thromboembolism** (blood clots), most commonly of the deeper veins in the legs. This risk has largely been eliminated by the lower doses of estrogen used in current formulations of oral contraceptive pills. In general, most women tolerate oral contraceptive pills well. The most common side effects include nausea/vomiting, increased breast sensitivity, headache, spotting or breakthrough bleeding, swelling of leg veins, and with some, weight gain. These are often temporary effects that resolve after the first few months of treatment. There can also be a transient flare of inflammatory acne when oral contraceptive pill therapy is started (Table 22).

Glucocorticoids: Glucocorticoids, such as prednisone or dexamethasone, in low doses can suppress the adrenal production of androgens. They can be used in male or female patients who have an elevation of DHEAS in the serum associated with a decrease in levels of 11- or 12-hydroxylase. These are measured through blood tests. Glucocorticoids can also be used in cases of acute acne flares or in very severe cases of acne for a few weeks. Low-dose prednisone (2.5 or 5 mg) or dexamethasone (0.25 to 0.75 mg) can be given by mouth at

Thromboembolism
blood clots.

Table 22. Side Effects of Oral Contraceptive Pills

Nausea/vomiting
Breast tenderness
Headache
Spotting/breakthrough bleeding
Swelling of leg veins
Weight gain
Irritability/depression/mood swings

bedtime to suppress adrenal androgen production. Side effects include other unwanted signs of adrenal suppression and can be followed with specific tests every 2 to 3 months after treatment is started.

The combination of glucocorticoids and estrogens has been used in recalcitrant acne in women with excellent results. The doses of estrogens typically used, however, are higher than the typical dose of estrogen used in oral contraceptives.

Inhibiting androgen metabolism: 5-α-reductase inhibitors: No therapies are available that inhibit the local production of androgens within the sebaceous gland. An inhibitor of 5-α-reductase would block the local conversion of testosterone to dihydrotestosterone. Specific inhibitors of the type 15-α-reductase are being developed. This type of treatment is helpful in that they inhibit sebum production and are therefore helpful in the treatment of acne.

PART EIGHT

Procedures Done in the Doctor's Office

What procedures can be used to treat acne?

Are chemical peels safe?

What is dermabrasion?

More ...

83. What procedures can be used to treat acne?

There are a number of procedures done in a doctor's office to treat acne. These procedures include chemical peels, **microdermabrasion**, **dermabrasion**, laser and laser-like procedures, **cryotherapy** with either liquid nitrogen or CO_2 slush, and surgery to remove scars. Most of these procedures are considered to be "cosmetic," meaning that they are generally not covered under most insurance plans. These are some of the procedures that are done in the doctor's office: chemical peels, microdermabrasion, cryotherapy, electrocautery, dermabrasion, laser, and surgery.

The treatment that is right for you will depend on your skin type, how much scarring you have, how active your acne is, and how much you can spend on these treatments. Most of the treatments listed need to be done several times to get proper results, and maintenance treatments are necessary to have lasting improvement over time. The procedures are safe if done properly and can be done along with a topical or oral regimen to maximize your results. Your doctor will determine the appropriate regimen for you and will monitor your results.

Chemical peels are an increasingly popular treatment to treat acne and to minimize scarring from acne. Several different solutions are available for chemical peels, and they each have their advantages and disadvantages. This is a list of the most commonly used chemical peels:

- glycolic (α-hydroxy acid, fruit acid), s
- alicylic acid (β-hydroxy acid),
- Jessner's solution, and
- trichloroacetic acid.

Microderm abrasion

a skin-freshening technique that helps repair facial skin.

Dermabrasion

a technique to "refinish" the skin's top layers through a method of controlled surgical scraping.

Cryotherapy

a treatment in which surface skin lesions are frozen using liquid nitrogen, carbon dioxide "slush," or other cryogens.

84. Are chemical peels safe?

Chemical peels are an increasingly popular treatment to treat acne and to minimize scarring from acne. There are several different solutions available for chemical peels, and each has its advantages and disadvantages (as listed previously).

Light chemical peels (meaning that they do not penetrate beyond the upper layers of the skin) may be useful in acne patients to help correct surface scarring and hyperpigmentation. After a light or superficial chemical peel, the skin may stay red for a few hours and then return to normal. It is unusual and undesired to have blisters or areas of bleeding after a superficial chemical peel. There is typically no obvious peeling of the skin after these treatments, and thus, the word "peel" is a misnomer.

Peeling agents include α-hydroxy acids (glycolic acid), salicylic acid, and trichloroacetic acid. Salicylic acid may have anti-inflammatory effects. Salicylic acid is fat soluble and may penetrate into the sebum-heavy follicles more easily than the water-soluble α-hydroxy acids. This makes salicylic acid an especially useful agent in the treatment of acne. There is also usually more active peeling after a salicylic acid treatment than with glycolic acid.

Trichloroacetic acid can be used in strengths from 5% to approximately 20% to achieve a superficial peel. There is generally more active peeling that occurs after a trichloroacetic acid peel, and this treatment generally should be done by a qualified dermatologist because the strength of the peel varies depending on how it is applied, and there is some risk of scarring associated with deeper penetration of the acid.

85. What is dermabrasion?

In the process of dermabrasion, the upper and middle layers of the skin are removed in order to improve acne scarring. Important considerations need to be addressed before undergoing this type of procedure. Dermabrasion is ideal for people with types I–IV skin (see Table 23) who have superficial scars. Healing time is involved, and local anesthetic is a must because the procedure is otherwise very painful.

The very deep, pitted scars are not considered ideal for this type of treatment as the scars would end up deep and wide and would most likely be more obvious after the treatment, which is clearly not the goal. For these types of scars, the best treatment is either to try to fill them with either temporary fillers, such as collagen or Restylane, or with one of the more permanent fillers available on the market like Artecoll. Another method of treating the deep pits or "ice-pick" types of scars is called **punch grafting**. This technique involves using a

Punch grafting

a technique that uses a cookie-cutter type blade to punch out a scar, followed by adding skin from another site to fill in the hole.

Table 23. Different Skin Types

Skin Type	Unexposed Skin Color	Tanning History
I	Ivory white, pale white	Burns easily, never tans
II	White	Burns easily, tans minimally
III	White	Burns moderately, tans evenly
IV	Beige or lightly tanned	Burns minimally, tans easily
V	Moderate brown or tanned	Rarely burns, tans profusely
VI	Dark brown	Never burns, tans profusely

cookie-cutter type of blade to punch out the scar, followed by adding in skin taken from another site to fill in the hole. After this, dermabrasion can be done to smooth the edges.

86. What is the difference between microdermabrasion and dermabrasion? How many microdermabrasion treatments do I need? Do they really work?

Microdermabrasion is a procedure in which fine crystals are essentially blasted at the skin and then vacuumed back away from the skin. These two components help clean out the pores, again temporarily, and make the skin feel smoother. The upper layers of the skin are exfoliated off, which helps other treatments penetrate more evenly.

Usually a series of five to seven microdermabrasion treatments are done to get optimal results, followed by maintenance treatments every 6 to 8 weeks. No really good studies exist showing the benefits of microdermabrasion; however, plenty of anecdotal evidence suggests that it does help in the treatment of acne.

87. Is cryotherapy right for me?

Cryotherapy involves the use of liquid nitrogen or carbon dioxide slush to treat acne. These procedures are useful, but they require special storage containers and are becoming less popular as newer treatments become available. The goal of these treatments is to exfoliate localized areas of skin where the pimples are concentrated.

Some people love the way their skin looks after the treatments, but there is a risk of scarring, and storage of the materials is difficult which makes this treatment relatively uncommon. Liquid nitrogen is very cold; in fact, it is $-195°$ F, which means that it needs to be stored in a special container since it evaporates at room temperature. Generally, both liquid nitrogen and CO_2 slush are applied by the doctor to specific pimples. Immediately after the treatment the site can turn red and become a little swollen. This generally lasts anywhere from half an hour to a day. Then the pimple dries up and exfoliates off with washing over the next few days or so. Sometimes the doctor will apply a very light layer of the cryogen to the entire face for a general peel. The skin usually turns red and then peels over the next week. Sometimes the peeling process is not noted as obvious peeling of the skin, but the skin looks smoother and feels softer to the touch.

88. What is electrocautery?

Electrocautery is the use of an electric current that is converted into heat and passed through a fine tip. It can be useful in a limited number of circumstances in the treatment of acne and is not often used. The heat applied directly to the acne lesion exfoliates the skin and kills the bacteria. It is also sometimes used to open whiteheads so the contents can then be extracted to clear the lesion. There is a risk of scarring from this treatment, which is one reason it is not considered a main treatment for acne.

89. What is the difference between laser and intense pulsed light treatments?

Laser stands for "light amplification by stimulated emission of radiation." Laser energy can be provided by various sources, from a gas to a liquid to a solid.

Electrocautery
the use of an electric current that is converted into heat and passed through a fine tip.

These energy sources allow for specific wavelengths of light to be intensified and directed through a column. We select the wavelength of light from our understanding of how those wavelengths are absorbed by the skin. We know that the longer the wavelength, the deeper the light penetrates. We also know that there are specific elements in the skin that prefer certain wavelengths of light.

In this way, we can target only the sebaceous glands or melanin high up in the skin or deeper within the skin. We can target water in the skin or various components of blood vessels within the skin. In this way, we can choose to heat and damage the skin in very specific ways without damaging surrounding skin tissue so that in the process of healing the skin will look clear and healthy—without acne or broken blood vessels or brown spots or even wrinkles.

Intense pulsed light devices are similar to lasers in that they can selectively target specific elements in the skin using specific wavelengths of light; however, these devices use a wider range of wavelengths as opposed to only one single beam of light. This can be very useful in that a within a range of light you can very effectively target your source. The most important advances in laser and intense pulsed light technology have been understanding and expanding their uses in very specific ways.

In the past, CO_2 lasers were used to heat water within the skin. This would cause destruction of the upper layers of the skin and sometimes go even deeper. There was a 2- to 3-month healing time, after which there could still be redness for months, and then areas of the skin could appear darker or lighter than the adjacent skin. This type of treatment is still used to treat certain types of acne scarring; however, it is not recommended for the treatment of active acne, or within 6 months of taking oral isotretinoin.

The newer devices can target the source of the acne, such as the sebaceous gland, the *P. acnes* bacterium, or the blood vessels that supply the swelling and redness, without damaging the surrounding skin. In this way, treatments can be done over time without limiting the activities of the person being treated. No "down time," or at least very little down time, exists. This advance has made these devices more accessible and more useful in the treatment of many skin conditions. They are also much less painful than the earlier devices.

90. What laser/light treatments are available?

Recently, the FDA has approved several lasers and light systems for the treatment of acne. These are designed to target only inflammatory acne with active growth of *P. acnes*. They are not effective for people who have only blackheads or whiteheads. Treatment routines vary depending on the system used.

In August 2002, the ClearLight was the first device to get clearance from the FDA for the treatment of acne. This system uses high-intensity, narrow-band light in the violet-blue portion of the light spectrum, not laser energy, for the treatment of moderate to severe inflammatory acne. The device works by targeting the bacterium *P. acnes* by using high intensity light to excite specific elements of *P. acnes* and in turn destroys them without harming the surrounding tissue.

The results of a multicenter study looking at 120 patients with treatments twice a week for 4 weeks showed that 80% of patients who had mild to moderate papulopustular acne experienced an approximately 60% improvement after treatment ended and a 70% improvement 2 weeks after the last treatment. There was no damage to surrounding tissue, and there were no reports of patient discomfort during the testing period.

Ongoing studies are looking at different treatment parameters, such as once-a-week treatments for 6 weeks and other variations to get maximal results with minimal intrusion on lifestyle. This type of treatment is only effective in the inflammatory types of acne since it is targeting the *P. acnes* bacterium.

Next came the Smoothbeam. This system is a diode laser that has clearance to treat both acne and depressed scars caused by acne. This laser emits energy at 1450 nm. A multiyear study done at the Naval Medical Center in San Diego found that acne lesion counts were significantly lower after only one treatment and that patients had a reduction in lesions of more than 98% after four 20-minute laser sessions. In addition, they reported that patients also noted a 6-month remission of acne lesions after treatment.

The CoolTouch is a 1320-nm laser system that is approved for back acne and acne scars. This laser targets the sebaceous glands without damaging the skin's surface.

The latest laser to get FDA approval is the Nlite-V laser system. It is a 585-nm pulsed dye laser. It is has FDA approval for moderate inflammatory acne on the face. This laser emits a wavelength of yellow light that heats small blood vessels, encouraging healing and stimulating collagen production. According to a study done on 41 patients in London, patients noted a 50% improvement in acne lesion counts after one 5-minute treatment session. Results typically lasted for up to 3 months.

The OmniLux Blue is a new type of system that uses light-emitting diodes in the visible spectrum at 415 nm. It is approved to treat mild to moderate inflammatory acne. Patients usually receive eight, 20-minute light treatments over a period of 4 weeks. In the studies done for FDA approval, 28% of patients in the study achieved optimum clearance at 4 weeks after treatment (average clearance was 76%); 55% had optimum clearance at 2 months (average clearance was 71%), and 17% had optimum clearance at 3 months (average clearance was 73%). Treatment was tolerated well.

The LuxV is an intense pulsed light-based system that is also approved for inflammatory acne.

The CO_2 and erbium lasers are known as "ablative" lasers in that they heat up larger areas of the skin and can have a significant amount of healing or down time associated with them. These are generally used to treat certain types of acne scars that are not very deep. They are more commonly used to treat signs of sun damage and wrinkles.

Radiofrequency energy is produced by an electrical current instead of a light source. It is not scattered by tissue or absorbed by melanin, making it safer for patients

Table 24.   Laser and Related Procedures

Laser
- OmniLux—blue light
- OmniLux Revive—red light
- Smoothbeam
- Aura (KTP—green light)
- CoolTouch
- Nlite-V
- CO_2
- Erbium

Intense pulsed light
- ClearLight

Light-emitting diodes
- OmniLux Blue

Radiofrequency
- Aurora

Experimental
- Pulsed dye therapy

with darker skin types. This type of energy also penetrates more deeply through the skin (Table 24).

91. How many treatments do I need?

The number of treatment sessions required to achieve results depends on the system used and the severity of acne at the start of treatment. Also, there are almost always maintenance treatments that are required to minimize acne flare-ups. Most insurance companies are either not covering the cost of laser/intense pulsed light treatments or are covering them for a specific number of treatments. It is important to check with your insurance company to make sure that you will be covered for the treatments or be prepared to discuss the fees with your doctor's office to make sure that you want to proceed.

92. How long does it take to see results?

Results from laser/intense pulsed light treatments can occur from 1 day to 1 month after starting treatment, depending on the system used and the severity of acne at the onset of treatment.

93. As an African-American woman, is laser safe for my skin type?

Technological advances are making laser treatments for acne safer for darker skin types (Table 23). Although acne is a common concern in people with darker skin, lasers have been avoided for acne treatment on darker skin because of the risk of potentially disfiguring complications such as acne scarring, keloids, and skin discoloration. There are some treatments, using both lasers and intense pulsed light devices, that are being tested for darker skin and that seem to show promising results for acne on the face and on the chest and back. As with other skin types, maintenance treatments are usually needed to minimize the recurrence of acne.

Lasers and intense pulsed light devices being used to treat acne in people with darker skin include the ClearLight (blue: 405 to 420 nm), the Aura laser (532-nm KTP laser, green light), and Aurora (intense pulsed light/radiofrequency combination device).

94. Can I do laser treatments while I am doing other oral/topical treatments?

Laser and intense pulsed light treatment are often combined with other, mostly topical, treatments for acne. When the procedures are completed, the topical treatments are continued as maintenance therapy to prevent the recurrence of acne. In general, retinoids are stopped for approximately 4 to 5 days before a laser/intense pulsed light treatment and then restarted 3 to 4 days after the treatment. Other medications such as topical antibiotics or BP may be stopped for 1 to 2 days around the procedure depending on the skin sensitivity. Make sure to review all of your medications with your doctor prior to any procedure so you are aware of your level of sensitivity.

PART NINE

Other Treatments/ Experimental Methods

Are herbal supplements safe for acne?
Do they work for acne?

How does photodynamic therapy work?

How do I know if a treatment I heard
about in the media will work?

More ...

95. Are herbal supplements safe for acne? Do they work for acne?

Oral herbal supplements are becoming more popular and are used in the treatment of nearly every condition known to humans. The problem with herbal supplements is that they are basically drugs that are not regulated. It is hard to know the exact ingredients being used and the concentrations of the ingredients in any given bottle. The advice here is to be very cautious before trying any untested medication or supplement.

96. How does photodynamic therapy work?

Once a staple of acne treatment, older ultraviolet light treatments are now known to provide only transient improvement, and prolonged use, especially of ultraviolet A, may worsen comedonal acne. Also, the increased risk of skin cancer and photoaging makes it an even less desirable therapy. A relatively new treatment, called photodynamic therapy, which uses a combination of a drug called 5-amino levulinic acid (ALA) and blue light or mixed blue and red light, is successfully being tapped to treat moderate to severe acne.

The dermatologist applies the 5-amino levulinic acid to the affected areas for about 15 to 30 minutes and then uses either a pulsed light device or pulsed dye laser to activate the areas where the 5-amino levulinic acid was applied. The results may have significant promise for treating the more severe forms of acne and are also being used to treat certain types of skin cancer.

97. How do I know if a treatment I heard about in the media will work?

Because acne is such a common condition, some are trying to promote treatments that may or may not be effective. This can be seen from the many ads and "too-good-to-be-true" claims, aimed mostly at teenagers who will try nearly anything to get "perfect" skin. On the other side, there have been many excellent topical and system drugs developed for the treatment of acne over the past 25 years. There has been continued improvement in the design of clinical trials with outcomes that provide excellent new therapies. Advances in medicine occur fairly rapidly, and new treatments are always on the horizon. The mission of the dermatologist is to provide safe treatments that are based on sound scientific evidence. Speak with your dermatologist about new over-the-counter or prescription treatments you hear or read about. I have many patients who bring in magazine and newspaper articles for my evaluation.

98. What acne treatments are now being evaluated?

Atrisone, a new topical gel, which contains a medicine called Dapsone (avlosulfon, an anti-infection agent), is believed to be a potent antibacterial and anti-inflammatory. This means it should help in both reducing the number of acne lesions and helping to decrease the redness associated with existing acne lesions.

Oral Dapsone was initially used as a treatment for malaria. It has since also been used for a variety of dermatologic and other medical conditions with sometimes excellent results. It can have serious side effects when taken by mouth and would therefore not be ideal for the treatment of acne; however, the topical form has been shown to be safe and is now being tested for efficacy in the treatment of acne. Dapsone can also be used with other topical or oral medications in the treatment of acne. This drug is now in phase III trials and should be available within the next few years.

A new topical drug is being developed and tested by Helix BioMedix, Inc. The working name of the product is HB64. From the results they have available to date, 40% of the study participants said that it helped greatly. Forty-five percent said it helped somewhat, and 15% said they were neither better nor worse. Also, 65% of the participants noted that this new gel performed better than other gel prescription products they had used, with only 10% saying that it worked worse. This new drug is seeking an indication for the treatment of mild to moderate acne.

Connectics Corp. has completed phase III testing on a new formulation of clindamycin 1% in a patented foam delivery system. It was shown to be as good as or better than the other clindamycin formulations on the market, and it gives the user one more choice in the treatment of his or her acne. Look for this new drug to be on the market very soon. There is also a new combination drug coming that contains clindamycin with tretinoin .025%, again going with the idea that most of us want as simple and complete a routine as possible.

99. Are any ongoing studies regarding acne taking place?

A good place to start is your local teaching hospital. You can call the dermatology clinic and ask whether any studies are currently underway and find out whether you are eligible. Also, as an excellent resource for acne and for nearly every question regarding the skin, you can look on the American Academy of Dermatology Web site for further information.

100. Where do I go for more information?

There are many resources available to provide information about acne treatment. A selection of the best such resources is listed in the Appendix that follows.

Organizations

American Academy of Dermatology
P.O. Box 4014
Schaumburg, IL 60168-4014
Phone: 847-330-0230
Fax: 847-330-0050
Web site: *www.aad.org*

The AAD Washington Office:
American Academy of Dermatology
1350 I St. NW, Suite 870
Washington, DC 20005-4355
Phone: 202-842-3555
Fax: 202-842-4355

U. S. Food and Drug Administration
5600 Fishers Lane
Rockville, MD 20857-0001
Main FDA number: 1-888-INFO-FDA (1-888-463-6332)
Drug Information Number: 301-827-4570 (8:00 am–4:30 pm Eastern Time)
Web sites:
   Main site: *www.fda.gov*
   Center for Drug Evaluation and Research: *www.fda.gov/cder/index.html*
   ASDSAccutane info: *www.fda.gov/cder/drug/infopage/accutane/*

Web Sites

Face facts.com
Medlineplus.com
Myclearskin.com

Glossary

Acnegenic: Products that induce inflammatory lesions (e.g. papules, pustules) to form. This reaction is a type of follicular irritant contact skin reaction that usually occurs within 2 to 3 days of using the product.

Acne excoriée: Acne that has been picked at or scratched repeatedly.

Acne vulgaris: The medical name for acne.

Aesthetician: A person trained to improve the appearance of skin through facial massage, application of skincare products or cosmetics, heat wraps, and similar techniques that affect only the skin surface.

α-hydroxy acids: Naturally occurring acids, derived from the sugars in particular plants, that are sometimes used in skin care products to promote turnover of dead skin cells.

Androgens: A class of hormones including testosterone and DHEAS. They cause the sebaceous gland to enlarge and produce more sebum, which is an important factor in the causation of acne.

Antibiotics: A large category of drugs that target bacteria.

Antioxidants: A substance that binds to free radicals, which can damage skin cells, in order to prevent such damage.

Azelaic acid: a natural material produced by a yeast that is used as a topical treatment for mild to moderate acne.

Basal cell carcinoma: A form of skin cancer affecting the cells at the bottom layer of the skin.

Benzoyl peroxide: An antiseptic commonly used topically in the treatment of acne. It does not induce bacterial resistance.

Biopsy: Collection of a tissue sample for laboratory examination, usually in cases where cancer or similar disease is suspected.

Blackheads: A type of acne that does not contain active bacteria. The contents of the follicle have turned black after exposure to oxygen. Also called **open comedo**.

Cataract: An opacity in the eye that obstructs vision. Cataracts are usually caused by UV exposure, diseases such as diabetes, or simple aging.

Chemical peels: The application of one or more chemicals to the face that "burn" off damaged cells.

Chlorhexidine: A broad-spectrum anti-microbial agent sometimes used in antibacterial soaps.

Clindamycin: An antibiotic effective against specific bacteria, sometimes used in acne treatment.

Closed comedo: A type of acne lesion that looks white. There is no active bacteria in this type of lesion.

Collagen: The main protein in connective tissue. It is responsible for the elasticity of the skin and plays a prominent role in development of scars.

Comedogenic: Products that induce open or closed comedones to form after about 2 to 3 weeks of use. Some products are labeled noncomedogenic, but this term is not specifically defined in the federal guidelines.

Contraindicated: A medication or procedure that should not be provided to or performed upon a patient with a particular illness because it will cause harm.

Corticosteroids: A group of anti-inflammatory drugs often used to inhibit allergic reactions or to treat severe inflammation.

Cryotherapy: A treatment in which surface skin lesions are frozen using liquid nitrogen, carbon dioxide "slush," or other cryogens.

Dermabrasion: A technique to "refinish" the skin's top layers through a method of controlled surgical scraping.

Dermatitis: Inflammation or irritation of the skin.

Electrocautery: The use of an electric current that is converted into heat and passed through a fine tip.

Endometrial cancer: The most common type of uterine cancer.

Erythromycin: An antibiotic commonly used to treat skin infections.

Esophagitis: Inflammation of the esophagus.

Esters: Oil-like emollients sometimes found in skin-care products.

Estrogen: Female sex hormone.

Exfoliation: The process of removing the upper layers of dead skin.

Exogenous ochronosis: Dark brown or black spots that occur in skin that has been treated with hydroquinones in large doses or for extended periods.

Facial: A process of various skin treatments, usually done by an aesthetician, with the intention of improving the skin.

Follicular plug: Blockage of the opening of the follicles. This is the one of the first steps in all types of acne.

Genetics: The factors that you inherit from your parents that determine many of your qualities and influence many more.

Glands: A group of cells that make a substance for use in the body.

Glycerin: A common additive in soaps and moisturizers to increase the moisture content of the skin.

Hair follicles: The unit that contains the hair and the roots of hair. It starts in the dermis and connects to the surface of the skin. There are hundreds of hair follicles on the face, most of which contain miniaturized hair that is not visible from the surface of the skin. Blockage of the follicle is called a follicular plug and is an early step in the process of all types of acne.

Hepatitis: Any disease featuring inflammation of the liver. Hepatitis can be caused by viral infection, alcohol or drug abuse, or exposure to certain toxins.

Heredity: The traits you get from your parents, such as tendency to acne, hair color, height, etc.

Hirsutism: The excessive growth of hair on a woman's face, torso and limbs, and is generally caused by increased androgens. It is a common sign of polycystic ovary syndrome in women.

Hormone: A chemical substance formed in one organ of the body, such as the adrenal gland, pituitary, or the ovary, etc., that is carried to another organ or tissue where it has a specific effect.

Hydroquinone: A class of chemicals that lighten the skin.

Hyperpigmentation: Darkening of skin caused by higher amounts of melanin in a particular spot.

Immune system: The collection of cells and structures in the body that fight disease or infection. White blood cells, lymph nodes, and lymph vessels are the primary components of the immune system.

Inflammatory acne: A class of acne where the main lesions are papules, and pustules, not comedones.

Intense pulsed light treatments: Treatments that incorporate a broad band of visible and near infrared wavelengths of light, blocking out other wavelengths. This produces broad bands of light that can penetrate various depths of skin and target both red and brown lesions. It also helps with collagen production, which makes skin look younger and more resilient.

Lasers: Machines that produce single bands of light, with different lasers being able to produce different single bands. These bands can be used to target various elements in the skin to help improve skin texture, tone and quality.

Lesion: A mark in the skin.

Lithium: A chemical element often used as a mood stabilizer.

Lupus erythematosus: An autoimmune disorder where antibodies are created against the body's own tissues, leading to a host of symptoms including a rash on the face.

Melasma: A skin condition presenting as brown patches on the face of adults.

Menstrual period: The monthly, cyclical bleeding cycle women experience when they are not pregnant. Irregularities in this cycle can indicate hormonal imbalance that can be an aggravating factor in acne.

Metabolism: Our bodies' natural energy requirements.

Microcomedo: The first stage of any type of acne lesion. It is so tiny as to be invisible.

Microdermabrasion: A skin-freshening technique that helps repair facial skin.

Open comedo: A type of acne lesion that looks black. There is no active bacteria in this type of lesion.

Oral contraceptive: Medications used by women to help prevent unwanted pregnancy. This category of medications is also now being very effectively used in the treatment of acne vulgaris in women. They decrease DHEAS and free testosterone levels and increase sex hormone-binding globulin.

Oxidation: Changes that occur after exposure to oxygen.

Parabens: A group of chemicals used as preservatives in cosmetics and as antibacterial agents in some antibacterial toothpastes.

Pilosebaceous unit: The grouping containing the hair follicle and attached sebaceous gland.

Polycystic ovary syndrome: A hormonal condition in women where the ovaries overproduce specific hormones. This can be manifest in the skin as increased and more severe acne, increased hair growth on the face, and hair loss on the scalp.

Pomade acne: A type of acne due to ingredients used in the hair. This acne is most commonly comedonal and is usually found on the forehead and temple regions of the face.

Pores: Openings of the follicles to the surface of the skin.

Prednisone: A corticosteroid commonly used to treat inflammation.

Prophylactically: A treatment or medication used in the absence of active disease, in order to prevent the condition from recurring.

Pseudotumor cerebri: Increased pressure build-up on the brain.

Puberty: Age at which sex hormones kick in, followed by specific changes, such as menses in girls and beard growth in boys.

Punch grafting: A technique that uses a cookie cutter-type blade to punch out a scar, followed by adding skin from another site to fill in the hole.

Retin-A: See Tretinoin.

Retinoids: Products, generally in the vitamin A family, that act at specific sites called retinoid acid receptors.

Retinol: Vitamin A.

Salicylic acid: Ingredient that helps exfoliate the upper layers of the skin. It is commonly found in over-the-counter acne treatment products.

Sebaceous glands: Oil-producing glands located in the deeper layers of the skin. They attach to the hair follicles and the oil travels up the follicle to end up on the surface of the skin.

Sebaceous hyperplasia: A condition caused by UVA exposure in which sebaceous glands grow and become lumpy and prominent in the skin.

Sebum: Oil produced by the sebaceous glands.

Squalene: Found in the sebum, squalene is an important precursor to androgen production.

Surfactants: Chemicals that lower the surface tension of a liquid, allowing easier spreading; they are often used in soaps and detergents.

Testosterone: A male sex hormone.

Tetracyclines: Class of antibiotics typically used in the treatment of acne vulgaris.

Thromboembolism: Blood clots.

Topical: A product that is used on the skin, such as a cream, lotion, or gel.

Tretinoin: Medication commonly used in the treatment of acne vulgaris. This compound is in the vitamin A family.

Triclosan: A potent wide-spectrum antibacterial and antifungal agent.

Ultraviolet radiation: Light emitted by the sun that can have damaging effects on skin.

Vehicle: The part of the product that holds the active ingredient, e.g., an oil, gel, or cream base into which the medication is added.

White blood cells: The body's main defense against infection.

Whiteheads: A type of acne lesion. White heads are white bumps in the skin that are closed to the surface. Also called **closed comedo**.

Index

A

Alpha-hydroxy acids. *see* Glycolic acid
Accutane (Isotretinoin, Sotret), 120–135
  and antibiotics, 132–133
  and birth defects, 83–84, 96, 128–129, 131
  dosing, 123–124, 125t, 134
  duration of treatment, 125, 134
  effectiveness of, 123
  indications for, 121
  initiating treatment, 124, 126t
  mechanisms of action, 122
  recurrence after, 135
  side effects, 112–113, 120–121,
    126–131, 131t
  things to avoid while taking, 131–132
  time to effectiveness, 125, 126–128
Acne cosmetica, 22t
Acne excoriée, 2, 22t, 29, 171
Acne instigators, 15t
Acne keloidalis, 22t
Acne, types of, 21–22, 22t
Acne vulgaris, 2, 22t, 171
Acnegenic, 59, 171
Adapalene (Differin), 76t, 93t
Adolescents, 24–26
Adult acne, 2, 54–57
  treating, 56–57
Aesthetician, 71, 171
African Americans, 41
  and laser treatments, 159, 160
Alcohol, and Accutane, 130
Alpha-hydroxy acid (glycolic acid), 76t,
  150, 151, 171
Alphaquin HP, 40t
American Academy of Dermatology, 167
Androgens, 18, 32–35, 33t, 56, 171
Antiandrogens, 144–145
Antibacterial soaps, 71

Antibiotics, 171
  oral, 24, 56
    and Accutane, 132–133
    combined with topical treatments, 96,
      99–100
    indications for, 104
    interaction with food, 116
    length treatment with, 114–115
    low-dose, 118
    mechanisms of action, 104, 105
    and oral contraceptives, 111–112
    during pregnancy, 85
    resistance to, 99–101, 107–109, 110
    side effects, 105–106, 110–111,
      112–113, 115
    and sun exposure, 113–114, 116–117
  selective action of, 109–111
  topical, 24, 60, 76t, 86, 89–91, 92t, 166
    during pregnancy, 96–97
Antioxidants, 39, 171
Antipsychotic medications, 57t
Artecoll, 152
Atrisone, 165–166
Aura laser system, 160
Aurora radiofrequency treatments, 158,
  159t, 160
Avita (tretinoin), 93t
Avlosulfon (Dapsone), 165–166
Azeliac acid (Azelex, Finacea), 76t, 171
  during pregnancy, 84, 85

B

Basal cell carcinoma, 114, 171
Benzoyl peroxide (BP), 24, 74, 76t, 88–91,
  171
  cleansers, 70–71
  combined with oral antibiotics, 96

combined with topical antibiotics, 60,
77, 89, 90–91
effectiveness of, 104
formulations, 90t
during pregnancy, 84, 85
and Retin-A, 77
vehicles for, 79
Beta-hydroxy acids. *see* Salicylic acid
Biopsy, 114, 171
Blackheads, 2, 8, 10, 171–172
Blood tests
for Accutane prescription, 126
for diagnosis, 67–68, 139–140, 139t

C

CO$_2$ lasers, 158
Cataracts, 97, 172
Causes, of acne, vi, vii, 7–8, 13–16, 15t,
Chemical peels, 133, 144, 150, 151, 172
Chlomadinone, 139t
Chlorhexidine, 71, 172
Chlormadinone acetate, 144
Chocolate, 44
Cleansers, 69, 70, 71, 72
ClearLight laser system, 156, 159t, 160
Clindamycin, 172
oral, 105t, 112
topical, 76t, 89, 90t, 166
Clinical trials, 166–167
Closed comedo (whitehead), 8, 172, 175
CO$_2$ lasers, 159t
Collagen, 52, 152, 172
Comedo, 30
closed, 7, 8, 172, 175
duration of, 27–28
extraction, 72
micro-, 7
Comedogenic, 17, 172
Comedonal acne, 22t
Connectics Corporation, 166
Contagiousness, 35–36
Contraceptives, oral, 174
and Accutane, 132
and antibiotics, 111–112
as cause of acne, 15, 28, 143–144
mechanisms of action, 143
side effects, 146, 147, 148t
for treatment of acne, 15, 57, 138–148
Contraindicated, 85, 172
CoolTouch laser system, 157, 159t
Corticosteroids, 57t, 97, 172

Cortisol, 33t, 35, 48–49
Cortisone, 98
Cosmetic treatments, 150
Cotrimoxazole, 105t
Cryotherapy, 150, 153–154, 172
Cyproterone acetate (CA), 139t, 144–145
Cysts, cystic acne, 12, 22t, 97–98
duration of cysts, 28

D

Dairy foods, 45–46
Dapsone (avlosulfon), 165–166
Depression, and Accutane, 124
Depression, and Isotretinoin (Accutane,
Sotret), 129
Dermabrasion, 150, 153, 172
Dermatitis, 69, 172
Dermatologists, 68–69
Desogestrel, 139t
Dexamethasone, 147, 148
DHA (dihydroxyacetone), 51–52
DHEAS (dehydroepiandrosterone sulfate),
33t, 34, 139t, 147
Diagnosis
blood tests, 67–68, 139–140
visiting the doctor, 68–69
Differin (adapalene), 76t, 93t
Dilantin (phenytoin), 57t
Doctor, visiting, 16, 25–26, 68–69
for Accutane prescription, 124
Doryx (doxycycline), 105t
Doxycycline, 85, 105t
low-dose (Periostat), 114, 118
and sun exposure, 112, 116–117
Drinking alcohol, and Accutane, 130
Drospirenone, 139t
Duration, of pimple, 27–28
Dynacin (minocycline), 105t

E

Eldoquin Forte, 40t
Electrocautery, 154, 172
Endometrial cancer, 146, 172
Epiquin, 40t
Erbium lasers, 158, 159t
Erythromycin, 105t, 172
during pregnancy, 84, 85, 96–97
topical, 76t, 84, 89, 90t
Esophagitis, 106, 172
Esters, 62, 172
Estrogens, 57t, 150, 172

for treatment, 138, 139t, 142–143
Exercise, 60–61
Exfoliation, 8, 19, 172
Exogenous ochronosis, 41, 172
Extraction, professional, 72

F

Facials, 21, 71–72, 172
FDA (Food and Drug Administration), 80
    drug safety ratings, 85, 86t
Finacea (azeliac acid), 76t
5-alpha-reductase inhibitors, 148
5-amino levulinic acid, 164
Flare-ups, 37
Flutamide, 139t, 146
Follicles, 14t
Follicular plug, 30, 172
Foods
    interaction with medications, 116
    as triggers, 44–45
Free testosterone, 139t
Freezing, chemical, 150, 153–154

G

Generic products, 80–82
Genetics, 6, 14, 15t, 17–18, 36–37, 172–173
Glands, 2, 173
Glucocorticoids, 138, 147, 148
Glycerin, 27
Glycolic acid (alpha-hydroxy acid), 41, 76t,
    150
Glyquin, 40t
Gonadotropin-releasing hormone ago-
    nists, 138, 139t

H

Hair, facial, 138, 150
Hair follicles, 2, 173
Hair loss, as side effect, 144
Hair removal, laser, 132–133
Haldol (haloperidal), 57t
HB64, 166
Helix BioMedix, 166
Hepatitis, 146, 173
Herbal supplements, 164
Heredity, 36–37, 173. *see also* Genetics
    definition, 18
Hirsutism, 138, 144, 150, 173
Hormonal therapy, 138–148. *see also* Con-
    traceptives, oral

for men, 147, 148
Hormones, 173
    as causative agents, 6, 15t, 17–18, 32–35,
        48–49
    evaluation of levels, 67–68
    medications containing, 57t
Hydrocortisone, 76t
Hydroquinones, 39-40, 76t, 173
Hydroxy acids, 76t. *see also* Glycolic acid
        (alpha-hydroxy acid); Salicylic acid
        (beta-hydroxy acid)
Hygiene, 46–47, 69–71
    and overwashing, 69
Hyperpigmentation, 38–39, 173

I

Immune system, 35, 173
Infantile acne, 23–24
Inflammatory acne, 4, 10–12, 11f, 22t, 105t,
        173
    treatment for
        antibiotics, 104–105
        lasers. *see* Laser treatments
        steroids, 97–98
Inflammatory cells, 14t
Insurance coverage, 158, 159
Intense pulsed light treatments, 21,
        154–161, 159t, 173
Iodine, 46
Isoniazid, 57t

J

Jessner's solution, 150

K

Keloids, 22t
Keratinocytes, 14t

L

Langerhans cells, 173
Laser treatments, 132–133, 150, 154–161
    ablative, 158
    combined with other treatments, 160–161
    course of treatment, 158, 159
    insurance coverage, 158, 159
    time to effectiveness, 159
    types of, 159t
Lasers, 21, 173
Lesions, 2, 173
Lithium, 57, 58t, 173

Lupus erythematosus, 112, 173
    and Accutane, 130
Lustra, Lustra AF, 40t
LuxV laser system, 158
Lymecycline, 105t

M

Macrolides, 105t
Makeup
    as cause, 58–60
    oil-free, 60
Medications
    as cause of acne, 6, 15t, 57–58, 58t
    for treatment. *see* Antibiotics, oral;
        Antibiotics, topical; Skin lighteners
Melanex, 40t
Melasma, 144, 150, 174
Menstrual period, 31–32, 174
Metabolism, 16, 174
Microcomedo, 7, 8–9, 174
Microdermabrasion, 150, 153, 174
Minocycline (Dynacin), 85, 105t, 112
Moisturizers, 87–88

N

National Institute of Musculoskeletal and
        Skin Diseases, 5f, 11f
Naval Medical Center, San Diego, 157
Neonatal acne, 22t, 23–24
Neosporin, 86
Nicomide, 117
Nlite-V laser system, 157, 159t
Nodular acne, 22t
    treating. *see* Accutane (Isotretinoin, Sotret)
Nodules, 10, 12
Noninflammatory acne, 9–10

O

Oil-free products, 60, 61–62
Oily skin, 31–32
OmniLux Blue laser system, 157–158, 159t
OmniLux Revive laser system, 159t
Open comedo (blackhead), 174
Osteoporosis, and Accutane, 129–130
Oxidation, 8, 174

P

Papules, 10
Parabens, 130–131, 142, 174
Period, menstrual, 31–32
Periostat (doxycycline), 105t, 114

Phenytoin, (Dilantin), 57t
Photodynamic therapy, 164
Picking, 8, 12–13, 28, 29–30, 64–65
Pilosibaceous unit, 5f, 17, 33–34, 174
Polycystic ovary syndrome, 32, 174
Pomade acne, 22t, 26–27, 174
Pores, vi, 174
    enlarged, 18–21
Potassium iodide, 57
Prednisone, 97, 138, 147, 148, 174
Pregnancy, treatment during, 83–85
    oral medications, 83–84
    safety categories, FDA, 86t
    topical medications, 96–97
Prevalence, of acne, vi, 5,
Prevention, 28
Prolactin, 139t
Prophylactic, prophylactically, 15, 174
Propionibacterium acnes, 4, 8, 12, 14t, 17, 35,
        36
    and exercise, 61
    and oral antibiotics, 104–105
    and sun exposure, 49–50
    and topical antibiotics, 86–87
Pseudomembranous colitis, 112
Pseudotumor cerebri, 113, 132–133, 174
Psychological impact, 6–7, 25–26
Puberty, 18, 174
Pulsed dye therapy, 159t
Punch grafting, 152–153, 174
Pustules, 10

Q

Quinine, 57t

R

Radiofrequency treatments, 158, 159t
Recurrance
    after Accutane treatment, 135
    in one spot, 66–67
Renova cream, 93t
Restylane, 152
Retin-A micro (tretinoin), 93t
Retin-A (tretinoin), 20, 24, 76t, 77. *see
        also* Retinoids
    and sun exposure, 113–114
Retinoids, 8, 41, 76t, 174
    combined with BP, 90
    and facial waxing, 95–96
    formulations, 93t
    and laser treatments, 161

mechanisms of action, 93–94
oral. *see* Accutane (isotretinoin, Sotret)
during pregnancy, 83
and skin irritation, 94, 95
Retinol, 32, 174
Roche corporation, 120–121

S

Salicylic acid (beta-hydroxy acid), 32, 76t,
150, 151, 174
Scarring, scars, 8, 28, 29, 30–31, 64–65
and sun exposure, 52
treating, 38–41, 151–152, 158
Sebaceous glands, 3, 14t, 16–18, 31, 174–175
and sex hormones, 32, 33, 34
Sebaceous hyperplasia, 113–114
Sebum, 4, 17, 18, 31–32, 175
and sex hormones, 32, 33
Self-confidence, 6–7
17-Hydroxyprogesterone, 139t
Skin
functions of, v–vi
structure of, 3–4, 3f, 5f, 7, 11
Skin color types, 160t
Skin lighteners, 39–41, 40t
Smoothbeam laser system, 157, 159t
Social impact, 6–7
Solaquin Forte, 40t
Sotret (Isotretinoin), 83–84
Spironolactone, 139t, 144–146
Steroid acne, 22t, 97–98
Steroids, 57t, 97–98
Stress, 14, 15–16, 47–50
and hormones, 28, 32, 35, 48–49
managing, 49–50
Stress hormones, 33t
Studies, clinical, 166–167
Sulfonamides, 105t
Sun exposure, 50–53
and antibiotics, 112, 116–117
and enlarged pores, 19, 20
and retinoids, 95
and scarring, 51
and ultraviolet radiation, 51–52

Sunscreen, 53–54
Surfactants, 47, 175
System to Monitor Accutane-Related Ter-
atogenicity (S. M. A. R. T), 84

T

T zone, 2, 31
Tanning creams, sunless, 52–53
Tanning lotions, 52–53
Tanning salons, 50–53, 113–114
Tazarotene, 93t
Tazorac, 76t
Teens, 24–26
and parental attitudes, 25–26, 44
Teeth, antibiotic effects on, 115
Testosterone, 33t, 34, 35, 57t, 139t, 175
Tetracyclines, 24, 85, 105t, 175
administration, 116
effects on teeth, 115
and pregnancy, 96
Thromboembolism, 147, 175
Tiluma, 40t
Topical, definition, 14, 175
Topical treatments, 14, 15, 76t
combined with antibiotics, 99–100
over-the-counter, 74
prescription, 74–75
vehicles for, 78–80
Treatments
brand name vs. generic products, 80–82
compliance with, 77, 87, 94, 101, 105–107
developing resistance to, 99
length of time to effectiveness, 75, 77,
82–83
planning, 13, 21, 64–66
and teens, 25–26
variety of, 77–78
Tretinoin (Retin-A), 24, 93, 94t, 175
Trichloroacetic acid, 150, 151
Triclosan, 71, 175
Triggers, of flare-ups, 37, 44–45
Trimethoprim, 85
Trimethoprim/sulfamethoxazole
(Bactrim), 105t

U

Ultraviolet radiation, 51–52, 113, 164, 175

V

Vehicles, for topical treatments, 78–80, 175
Vision changes, and Accutane, 130
Vitamin A, 32. *see also* Retinoids
Vitamin therapy, 117

W

Waxing, facial, 95–96, 132
White blood cells, 4, 175
Whiteheads (closed comedo), 2, 8, 9–10, 175

Z

Zinc therapy, 117